Barbara O'Neill's Teachings On Natural Healing

Harness Nature's Power Self-Healing | Effective Strategies
for Healing, Vitality, and a Holistic Approach to Wellness

Laura Peterson Clark

Copyright

Disclaimer

The information provided in this book is for educational purposes only and is not intended as medical advice. The content is not intended to diagnose, treat, cure, or prevent any disease. Always consult with a qualified healthcare professional before beginning any new health regimen or if you have any questions regarding a medical condition.

The author has made every effort to ensure that the information in this book was correct at the time of publication. However, the author does not assume and hereby disclaims any liability to any party for any loss, damage, or disruption caused by errors or omissions, whether such errors or omissions result from negligence, accident, or any other cause.

Trademarks

All trademarks, service marks, product names, and logos appearing in this book are the property of their respective owners. Use of these marks does not imply any affiliation with or endorsement by the trademark holders.

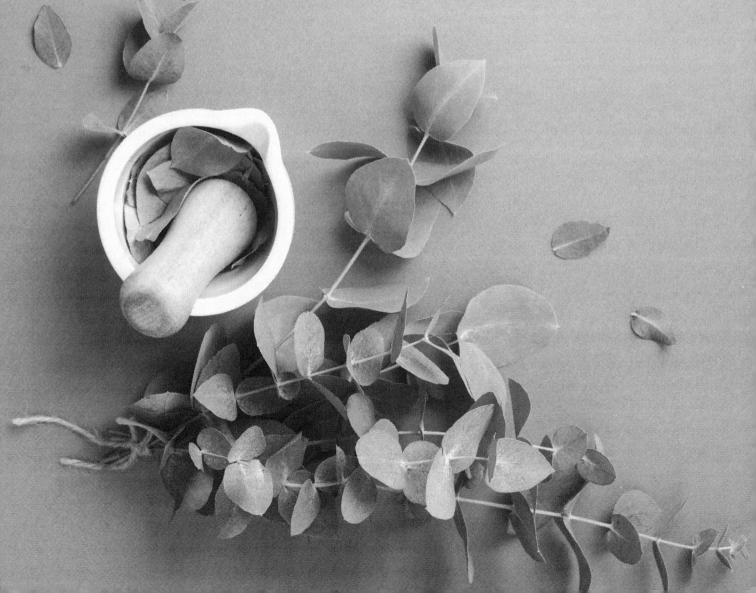

Table of Contents

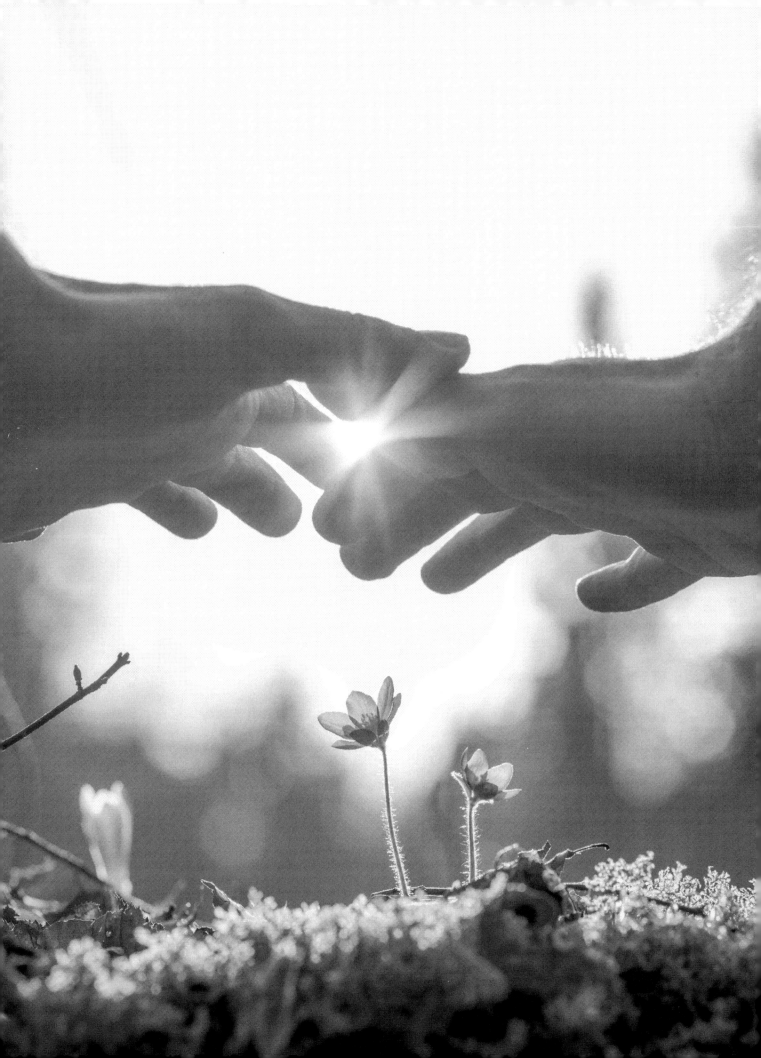

Embracing the Path of Natural Healing

Introduction to Natural Healing

In the modern world, the pace of life has become exceedingly fast, often at the expense of our health and well-being. Many individuals find themselves trapped in a cycle of stress, poor diet, and over-reliance on pharmaceutical interventions that may treat symptoms but do not address the root causes of illness. This growing dissatisfaction with conventional medicine has led to a resurgence in interest in natural healing, a holistic approach that emphasizes the body's inherent ability to heal itself when given the proper support. Natural healing is not a new concept; it is rooted in ancient practices that have been honed and refined over centuries across diverse cultures.

Natural healing, also known as holistic healing, is a comprehensive approach that encompasses a variety of practices aimed at promoting health and preventing disease by aligning the body, mind, and spirit with the natural rhythms of life. At its core, natural healing is based on the principle that the body has an innate ability to heal itself, provided it is given the right tools and environment. These tools include proper nutrition, herbal medicine, physical activity, mental well-being, and environmental harmony.

One of the key aspects of natural healing is the use of **herbal medicine**, which har-nesses the medicinal properties of plants to support and enhance the body's healing processes. Herbs have been used for millennia by various cultures around the world, including the Egyptians, Greeks, Chinese, and Native Americans. Each culture developed its own system of herbal medicine based on the plants available to them and their unique philosophies of health and disease.

For instance, Traditional Chinese Medicine (TCM) views illness as an imbalance in the body's energy, or qi, and uses herbs to restore this balance. Similarly, Ayurveda, the ancient healing system of India, employs a vast array of herbs to balance the body's three doshas (vata, pitta, and kapha) and maintain overall health. These ancient practices have laid the foundation for modern herbal medicine, which continues to explore and validate the therapeutic potentials of plants through scientific research.

In addition to herbal medicine, natural healing encompasses **nutritional therapy**, which emphasizes the importance of a balanced diet rich in whole foods, superfoods, and adequate hydration. Nutritional therapy is not just about preventing deficiencies but also about optimizing the body's functions. For example, a diet high in antioxidants, such as those found in berries and leafy greens, can help reduce oxidative stress and inflammation, which are underlying factors in many chronic diseases.

Another critical component of natural healing is **physical activity**. Regular exercise is essential for maintaining cardiovascular health, muscular strength, and overall vitality. Practices such as yoga and tai chi are particularly beneficial as they combine physical movement with mindfulness, promoting both physical and mental well-being. Exercise also supports the body's detoxification processes by enhancing lymphatic circulation and sweating.

Mental and emotional health are also integral to natural healing. Chronic stress and negative emotions can have profound effects on physical health, contributing to conditions such as hypertension, digestive disorders, and a weakened immune system. Natural healing advocates for practices that promote mental and emotional balance, such as meditation, mindfulness, and adequate rest. These practices help to calm the mind, reduce stress, and enhance the body's ability to heal.

Environmental factors play a significant role in natural healing. Our surroundings can either support or hinder our health. Exposure to toxins, pollutants, and a sedentary lifestyle can contribute to ill health, while a clean environment, rich in natural light and fresh air, can enhance well-being. Natural healing encourages individuals to create living spaces that are harmonious with nature, incorporating elements such as plants, natural light, and clean air.

A real-world example of the efficacy of natural healing can be seen in the case of Sarah, a middle-aged woman who suffered from chronic migraines and digestive issues. After years of relying on prescription medications with limited success and significant side effects, Sarah decided to explore natural healing. She consulted with a naturopath who recommended a comprehensive plan that included dietary changes, herbal supplements, regular exercise, and stress reduction techniques. Over several months, Sarah's migraines became less frequent and severe, and her digestive issues improved significantly. By addressing the root causes of her health problems through natural means, Sarah was able to achieve lasting relief and a better quality of life.

Natural healing is not just about treating illness; it is about nurturing a lifestyle that promotes overall health and prevents disease. It empowers individuals to take an active role in their health, making informed decisions that align with their body's natural needs. This holistic approach recognizes that health is a dynamic state of balance and harmony, requiring ongoing care and attention.

Barbara O'Neill's Journey and Philosophy

Barbara O'Neill's journey into the realm of natural healing is a story of transformation, dedication, and unwavering belief in the body's inherent ability to heal itself. Her philosophy is deeply rooted in the principles of holistic health, which emphasize the interconnectedness of the body, mind, and spirit. Her teachings, inspired by years of study and personal experience, have empowered countless individuals to take control of their health through natural means.

Barbara O'Neill began her career in the healthcare industry, initially working within the conventional medical system. However, she quickly became disillusioned with the limitations of this approach, particularly its tendency to treat symptoms rather than addressing the root causes of illness. This realization led her to explore alternative therapies, and she soon discovered the profound potential of natural healing. Her personal experiences with health challenges, combined with her professional background, fueled her passion for holistic health and inspired her to pursue extensive training in naturopathy and herbal medicine.

O'Neill's philosophy is centered on the belief that the body is a self-regulating organism capable of maintaining health and healing itself when provided with the right conditions. This concept, known as the vis medicatrix naturae, or the healing power of nature, is a cornerstone of naturopathic medicine. She advocates for a holistic approach that considers the physical, emotional, and environmental factors influencing health. According to O'Neill, true healing can only occur when all aspects of an individual's life are in harmony.

One of the key tenets of Barbara O'Neill's philosophy is the importance of nutrition in maintaining health and preventing disease. She emphasizes the role of a balanced diet rich in whole foods, organic produce, and natural supplements. Her dietary recommendations often include a focus on raw foods, juices, and nutrient-dense superfoods, which she believes provide the body with the essential vitamins, minerals, and enzymes needed for optimal functioning. O'Neill's approach to nutrition is not just about eating healthily but also about understanding how different foods affect the body and using this knowledge to make informed dietary choices.

Her teachings also highlight the significance of detoxification in maintaining health. O'Neill asserts that modern lifestyles expose individuals to a myriad of toxins, from processed foods to environmental pollutants, which can overwhelm the body's natural detoxification mechanisms. She advocates for regular detoxification practices, such as fasting, juicing, and the use of specific herbs, to support the liver, kidneys, and other organs involved in eliminating toxins. These practices, she believes, are essential for preventing chronic diseases and maintaining overall vitality.

In addition to nutrition and detoxification, Barbara O'Neill places a strong emphasis on the therapeutic use of herbs. She believes that herbs offer a natural and effective way to support the body's healing processes. Her extensive knowledge of herbal medicine allows her to recommend specific herbs for various health conditions, from digestive disorders to hormonal imbalances. O'Neill encourages the use of whole plant extracts and preparations, which she argues are more effective and safer than isolated compounds because they preserve the natural synergy of the plant's constituents.

Barbara O'Neill's philosophy extends beyond physical health to encompass mental and emotional well-being. She recognizes the profound impact that stress, emotions, and mental states can have on physical health and advocates for practices that promote mental and emotional balance. Techniques such as meditation, mindfulness, and positive thinking are integral to her approach, as they help individuals manage stress and cultivate a sense of inner peace and resilience. O'Neill believes that emotional health is just as important as physical health and that true wellness can only be achieved when both are addressed.

Her teachings are also deeply influenced by her respect for the natural world and her commitment to sustainability. O'Neill advocates for the use of organic and sustainably sourced herbs and foods, emphasizing the importance of preserving the integrity and potency of natural medicines. She is a strong proponent of environmental stewardship, encouraging individuals to adopt practices that protect the planet while promoting personal health.

A real-world example of Barbara O'Neill's impact can be seen in the story of John, a man in his late forties who struggled with chronic fatigue and digestive issues. After years of conventional treatments that provided little relief, John attended one of O'Neill's workshops. Inspired by her teachings, he adopted a diet rich in raw foods and began using specific herbs recommended by O'Neill. Within a few months, John's energy levels improved significantly, and his digestive issues were greatly alleviated. This transformation was a testament to the power of O'Neill's holistic approach and her ability to empower individuals to take charge of their health.

The Importance of Holistic Health

A holistic approach to wellness is an all-encompassing method of achieving wellbeing that takes into account the entire individual, including the body, mind, spirit, and emotions, in order to achieve optimal health and balance. Holistic health seeks to address the underlying causes of health problems and to promote general well-being, in contrast to traditional medicine, which frequently focuses on treating certain symptoms or illnesses in isolation. In this approach, it is acknowledged that all areas of a person's life are interconnected, and that genuine healing necessitates a harmonious balance between all of these components.

One of the fundamental principles of holistic health is the belief in the body's inherent ability to heal itself. This self-healing capability is supported by providing the body with the right tools and conditions, including proper nutrition, regular physical activity, mental and emotional balance, and a supportive environment. Holistic health practitioners work to empower individuals to take an active role in their health, encouraging them to make lifestyle choices that promote long-term wellness.

Proper nutrition is a cornerstone of holistic health. A diet rich in whole, unprocessed foods provides the essential nutrients needed for the body to function optimally. This includes vitamins, minerals, antioxidants, and other phytonutrients that support the immune system, reduce inflammation, and promote cellular repair and regeneration. In holistic health, food is not just seen as fuel but as medicine that can prevent and treat disease.

As an illustration, consuming a diet that is abundant in antioxidants, which can be found in fruits, vegetables, nuts, and seeds, can assist in the fight against oxidative stress and reduce the chance of developing chronic diseases such as diabetes, cancer, and heart disease. Walnuts, flaxseeds, and fatty fish are all good sources of omega-3 fatty acids, which have anti-inflammatory qualities and can help promote cognitive function and heart health through their consumption. It is possible for individuals to strengthen their body's natural defenses and improve their general vitality by concentrating on foods that are rich in nutrients.

Holistic health also requires exercise. Regular exercise improves mental health and strengthens the heart, muscles, and bones. Yoga, tai chi, and Pilates use mindfulness and movement to relax, reduce tension, and clear the mind. Exercise boosts mood-boosting endorphins and regulates cortisol. Regular exercise improves fitness, mental health, and quality of life.

Mental and emotional health are integral to holistic health. Chronic stress, anxiety, and negative emotions can have detrimental effects on physical health, contributing to conditions such as hypertension, digestive disorders, and a weakened immune system. Holistic health emphasizes the importance of mental and emotional balance, using techniques such as meditation, mindfulness, and deep-breathing exercises to manage stress and promote a sense of inner peace. These practices help individuals develop resilience, improve their ability to cope with challenges, and foster a positive outlook on life.

A real-life example of the power of holistic health can be seen in the case of Emily, a woman in her early thirties who struggled with anxiety and digestive issues for years. After numerous visits to various specialists and a barrage of medications that offered only temporary relief, Emily decided to explore holistic health. She began practicing yoga and meditation daily, changed her diet to include more whole foods and fewer processed items, and started using herbal remedies such as chamomile and peppermint for their calming and digestive properties. Over time, Emily's anxiety levels decreased significantly, and her digestive issues improved. This transformation highlights the effectiveness of a holistic approach in addressing the root causes of health problems rather than merely alleviating symptoms.

Environmental factors also play a crucial role in holistic health. The environments in which we live and work can significantly impact our health and well-being. Exposure to toxins, pollutants, and a sedentary lifestyle can contribute to a range of health problems. Holistic health encourages individuals to create living and working spaces that are clean, safe, and in harmony with nature. This includes using non-toxic cleaning products, ensuring good ventilation, incorporating plants to improve air quality, and designing spaces that promote physical activity and relaxation.

In addition to the physical environment, the social environment is equally important. Strong social connections and a supportive community can enhance emotional well-being and provide a sense of belonging and purpose. Holistic health recognizes the importance of social interactions and encourages individuals to build and maintain meaningful relationships. Engaging in community activities, volunteering, and spending time with loved ones can foster a sense of connection and support that is vital for overall health.

Spirituality is equally important in holistic wellness. This does not entail following a religion, but acknowledging the relevance of spiritual practices that provide meaning, purpose, and connection to something higher. Meditation, prayer, and nature can calm the mind and bring happiness.

For one to successfully incorporate holistic health into their daily lives, they must make a commitment to making decisions that are mindful and that support all parts of their well-being. The adoption of good eating habits, the participation in regular physical exercise, the management of stress via the use of mindfulness and relaxation techniques, the creation of a healthy living environment, the cultivation of social relationships, and the growth of spiritual practices are all included in this consideration. Individuals are able to create a condition of balance and harmony that is beneficial to their long-term heath and resilience if they adopt a holistic approach to health care.

The importance of holistic health lies in its comprehensive and integrative approach to wellness. By addressing the interconnected aspects of physical, mental, emotional, and spiritual health, holistic health provides a framework for achieving optimal well-being. This approach empowers individuals to take charge of their health, make informed choices, and cultivate a lifestyle that promotes balance, vitality, and resilience. As the understanding and acceptance of holistic health continue to grow, more individuals can benefit from its transformative potential and enjoy a higher quality of life.

CHAPTER 1

Foundations of Natural Healing

1.1 Historical Context and Evolution of Natural Remedies

The use of natural remedies is as ancient as human civilization itself, deeply rooted in the knowledge and traditions of early societies. From the dawn of humanity, individuals have sought out plants and natural substances to heal their ailments, driven by an instinctive understanding of the natural world around them. The historical context and evolution of natural remedies provide a fascinating insight into how these practices have developed over millennia, influenced by cultural exchanges, scientific discoveries, and an enduring belief in the healing power of nature.

The origins of natural remedies can be traced back to prehistoric times, where early humans relied on their observations and experiences to identify plants with medicinal properties. Archaeological evidence suggests that as far back as 60,000 years ago, Neanderthals in what is now Iraq were using plants such as yarrow and chamomile, which are still valued for their therapeutic properties today. This early use of medicinal plants laid the foundation for the development of more sophisticated herbal practices.

As societies evolved, so too did their understanding of natural remedies. Ancient civilizations such as the Egyptians, Sumerians, and Babylonians documented their herbal knowledge on clay tablets and papyrus scrolls. The Ebers Papyrus, dating back to 1550 BCE, is one of the oldest known medical texts, detailing over 700 remedies and formulas used by the ancient Egyptians. These early records highlight the significance of plants like aloe vera, garlic, and myrrh in their healing practices.

In Ancient Greece, the practice of natural healing was further refined by renowned figures such as Hippocrates, often referred to as the "Father of Medicine." Hippocrates emphasized the importance of diet, lifestyle, and natural therapies in maintaining health, a philosophy encapsulated in his famous adage, "Let food be thy medicine and medicine be thy food." His works, along with those of Dioscorides, whose seminal text "De Materia Medica" became a cornerstone of herbal knowledge for centuries, underscored the critical role of natural remedies in early Western medicine.

Simultaneously, in the East, traditional Chinese medicine (TCM) was developing its own extensive pharmacopeia. Rooted in the concepts of yin and yang and the balance of qi (vital energy), TCM employed a variety of herbs to restore harmony within the body. The Shennong Ben Cao Jing, attributed to the mythical Emperor Shennong around 2000 BCE, is one of the earliest Chinese texts detailing the medicinal properties of herbs. Similarly, Ayurveda, the ancient Indian system of medicine, dating back over 5,000 years, utilized a comprehensive approach to healing that incorporated diet, herbal treatments, and spiritual practices. The Charaka Samhita and the Sushruta Samhita are seminal texts that continue to influence Ayurvedic practice today.

The Middle Ages saw the transmission of herbal knowledge through the writings of scholars in the Islamic world. Avicenna, a Persian polymath, wrote the "Canon of Medicine," which integrated Greek, Roman, and Islamic medical knowledge and included detailed descriptions of hundreds of medicinal plants. This era also witnessed the preservation and expansion of herbal knowledge in European monasteries, where monks cultivated medicinal gardens and transcribed ancient texts.

The Renaissance period marked a resurgence in the study of natural remedies, driven by increased exploration and the exchange of knowledge between different cultures. Herbalists like Paracelsus challenged traditional medical practices and promoted the use of plant-based remedies. The publication of herbals—books detailing the properties and uses of plants—became widespread, with notable works such as John Gerard's "Herball" and Nicholas Culpeper's "The English Physician." These texts not only cataloged native European plants but also incorporated knowledge of exotic species discovered through global exploration.

The 19th and early 20th centuries saw significant advancements in the scientific understanding of medicinal plants. The isolation of active compounds such as quinine from cinchona bark and salicylic acid from willow bark paved the way for the development of modern pharmaceuticals. However, this period also marked a shift towards synthetic drugs and a decline in the use of traditional herbal remedies. Despite this, the latter half of the 20th century witnessed a renewed interest in natural medicine, spurred by a growing awareness of the limitations and side effects of conventional treatments.

In contemporary times, the integration of traditional knowledge with modern scientific research has led to a greater appreciation of natural remedies. Herbal medicine is now recognized as a complementary and alternative approach within mainstream healthcare. Studies validating the efficacy of herbs like echinacea for immune support, turmeric for its anti-inflammatory properties, and St. John's wort for depression have bolstered the credibility of natural remedies.

One real-world example of the enduring relevance of natural remedies is the widespread use of turmeric in both traditional and modern medicine. In Ayurveda, turmeric has been used for centuries to treat a variety of conditions, including digestive disorders, skin diseases, and joint pain. Modern research has identified curcumin, the active compound in turmeric, as a potent anti-inflammatory and antioxidant. This has led to its incorporation into contemporary treatments for conditions such as arthritis and metabolic syndrome, demonstrating the seamless blend of ancient wisdom and modern science.

The evolution of natural remedies reflects humanity's enduring quest for health and well-being through the power of nature. From the earliest use of plants by prehistoric humans to the sophisticated herbal systems of ancient civilizations, and from the scientific breakthroughs of the Renaissance to the modern validation of traditional knowledge, natural remedies have continually adapted to meet the changing needs of society. This rich history underscores the importance of preserving and integrating traditional healing practices with contemporary medical advancements to promote holistic health and wellness.

1.2 Understanding the Body's Natural Healing Processes

The human body is an intricate and remarkably resilient organism, endowed with an innate ability to heal itself. This natural healing process is a fundamental principle of holistic health, emphasizing the importance of supporting and enhancing the body's inherent capacities. Understanding these processes involves delving into the physiological mechanisms that enable recovery and restoration, as well as the holistic practices that can facilitate and optimize these natural functions.

At the core of the body's natural healing processes is the principle of homeostasis—the ability of the body to maintain internal stability despite external changes. Homeostasis involves a complex interplay of various systems that work together to regulate and balance bodily functions. When homeostasis is disrupted, the body initiates healing mechanisms to restore balance and health.

The body's immune system is one of the most important components of the natural healing processes that occur within the body. The immune system is a complex network of cells, tissues, and organs that work together to protect the body from pathogens: bacteria, viruses, and other foreign invaders. The immune system is responsible for defending the body against these infections. The innate immune system, which offers a defense that is immediate but not particular, and the adaptive immune system, which offers a reaction that is more targeted and lasts for a longer period of time, are the two primary components that make up this system.

The initial line of protection is the innate immune system. Skin, mucous membranes, phagocytes, and natural killer cells are its defenses. When a pathogen breaks these barriers, the innate immune system quickly neutralizes it. Innate responses like inflammation and clotting protect infection and start healing after a cut.

On the other hand, the adaptive immune system employs lymphocytes (B cells and T cells) that are able to identify particular antigens. This system is more specialized than the innate immune system. When a pathogen is introduced into the body, the adaptive immune system generates memory cells that remember the pathogen. These memory cells allow the immune system to provide responses that are both more rapid and more effective in the event of repeat infections. This is the fundamental idea underpinning vaccinations, which are designed to excite the adaptive immune system in order to develop immunity without actually causing disease.

Inflammation is another crucial aspect of the body's natural healing processes. Although often perceived negatively, inflammation is a vital response to injury and infection. When tissues are damaged, the body releases chemicals that cause blood vessels to leak fluid into the tissues, resulting in swelling. This inflammatory response helps isolate the affected area, preventing the spread of infection and promoting healing. The increased blood flow brings immune cells and nutrients to the site of injury, facilitating tissue repair and regeneration.

For example, consider the healing of a sprained ankle. Initially, the area becomes swollen and painful due to the inflammatory response. This acute inflammation, though uncomfortable, is essential for healing as it brings necessary cells and nutrients to repair the damaged ligaments. As the healing progresses, inflammation subsides, and the tissue begins to regenerate and strengthen.

Cell regeneration and repair are fundamental to the body's ability to heal. Different tissues have varying capacities for regeneration. For instance, skin cells regenerate rapidly, which is why minor cuts and abrasions heal quickly. In contrast, nerve cells in the central nervous system have limited regenerative abilities, which is why spinal cord injuries often result in long-term damage. Stem cells play a crucial role in regeneration, as they have the unique ability to develop into various types of cells needed for repair.

Detoxification is another key process in natural healing. The body constantly encounters toxins from the environment, food, and metabolic processes. Organs such as the liver, kidneys, lungs, and skin work tirelessly to detoxify the body, converting harmful substances into less toxic forms and excreting them. The liver, for instance, processes drugs and chemicals, rendering them harmless and facilitating their elimination through urine or bile. Supporting these detoxification pathways through proper nutrition, hydration, and lifestyle practices can enhance the body's ability to cleanse itself and maintain health.

The mental and emotional well-being of an individual has a considerable impact on the natural healing processes of the body. Homeostasis can be disrupted and immune function can be impaired when chronic stress and negative emotions are present. Cortisol and other stress hormones are released by the body in reaction to stress. When these hormones are increased for extended periods of time, they can cause inflammation and a diminished immunological response. Meditation, mindfulness, and exercises that focus on deep breathing are all practices that can assist in the management of stress and the promotion of emotional equilibrium, so making the body's inherent healing capacities more effective.

Nutrition plays a pivotal role in the body's healing processes. Nutrient-rich foods provide the vitamins, minerals, antioxidants, and other compounds necessary for cellular repair, immune function, and overall health. For instance, vitamin C is essential for collagen synthesis, which is crucial for wound healing. Zinc supports immune function and tissue repair, while antioxidants from fruits and vegetables protect cells from damage by free radicals.

Herbal medicine offers valuable support for the body's natural healing processes. Herbs such as echinacea, elderberry, and garlic can boost immune function, while turmeric and ginger have potent anti-inflammatory properties. Adaptogenic herbs like ashwagandha and rhodiola can help the body adapt to stress, enhancing resilience and promoting overall well-being. By incorporating these herbs into their diet or using them as supplements, individuals can support their body's natural healing processes.

A real-world example of the body's natural healing processes can be seen in the recovery from the common cold. When exposed to the cold virus, the immune system responds by producing antibodies and activating immune cells to fight the infection. Symptoms such as a runny nose, cough, and fever are manifestations of the immune response. The inflammation and mucus production help trap and expel the virus, while the fever creates an inhospitable environment for viral replication. With rest, proper nutrition, and hydration, the body typically overcomes the infection within a week or two, showcasing its remarkable self-healing abilities.

1.3 The Role of Mind, Body, and Spirit in Wellness

The concept of holistic wellness emphasizes the interconnection between the mind, body, and spirit, recognizing that optimal health can only be achieved when all three components are in balance. This comprehensive approach to health and well-being is foundational in natural healing practices, which aim to treat the whole person rather than just addressing isolated symptoms. Understanding the role of mind, body, and spirit in wellness involves exploring how these elements interact and influence one another, and how integrating them into a cohesive wellness strategy can lead to profound improvements in health.

One of the most important factors in total wellbeing is the **mind**, which has an impact on both one's physical health and their emotional well-being. The concept of mental health comprises a wide range of aspects, such as cognitive function, emotional control, and psychological resilience. Stress, anxiety, and negative thought patterns that persist over time can have a significant impact on one's physical health, leading to illnesses such as high blood pressure, digestive issues, and a compromised immune system. On the other hand, having a pleasant mental state can also improve one's physical health, strengthen one's immune system, and increase one's longevity.

Stress is one way the mind impacts the body. Cortisol and adrenaline are released when a threat is perceived. In preparation for a "fight or flight" response, these hormones raise heart rate, blood pressure, and energy. In acute settings, the stress response is useful, but chronic activation can cause cardiovascular disease, metabolic abnormalities, and immunological dysfunction. Mindfulness, meditation, and cognitive-behavioral therapy can reduce stress and boost mental health.

A real-world example of the mind-body connection can be seen in the practice of **mindfulness meditation**. Research has shown that regular meditation can reduce stress, lower blood pressure, and improve immune function. In one study, participants who practiced mindfulness meditation for eight weeks exhibited significant reductions in markers of inflammation and increased activity in brain regions associated with positive emotional states. This illustrates how cultivating a positive mental state can lead to tangible improvements in physical health.

The **body** is the physical aspect of wellness, encompassing all the biological systems and processes that sustain life. Physical health is influenced by factors such as nutrition, exercise, sleep, and the presence or absence of disease. Maintaining physical health is essential for overall well-being, as it provides the foundation upon which mental and spiritual health can flourish.

Proper **nutrition** is fundamental to physical health, providing the body with the essential nutrients needed for energy production, cellular repair, and overall functioning. A diet rich in whole, unprocessed foods supports the body's natural healing processes and helps prevent chronic diseases. For example, omega-3 fatty acids found in fatty fish and flaxseeds have anti-inflammatory properties that can protect against heart disease, while antioxidants in fruits and vegetables can reduce oxidative stress and lower the risk of cancer.

Regular **physical activity** is another crucial component of physical health. Exercise strengthens the cardiovascular system, enhances muscular and skeletal health, and promotes metabolic efficiency. Activities such as yoga and tai chi also incorporate elements of mindfulness and breath control, bridging the gap between physical and mental health. Exercise releases endorphins, which are natural mood elevators, and can improve sleep quality, reduce anxiety, and boost overall energy levels.

To maintain physical health, it is necessary to get enough sleep since it enables the body to repair and replenish itself. A lack of sleep over an extended period of time has been linked to a variety of health issues, including as obesity, diabetes, cardiovascular disease, and decreased cognitive performance. The establishment of good sleep hygiene, which includes the maintenance of a regular sleep schedule and the creation of a sleep environment that is more conducive to rest, can be beneficial to overall wellness.

The **spirit** represents the non-physical aspect of wellness, encompassing elements such as purpose, meaning, and connection to something greater than oneself. Spiritual health can be nurtured through practices that promote self-awareness, compassion, and a sense of interconnectedness. This can include religious or spiritual practices, time spent in nature, creative expression, and community involvement.

A strong spiritual foundation can provide individuals with a sense of purpose and direction, enhancing resilience and coping abilities in the face of life's challenges. For instance, engaging in **nature-based activities** such as hiking or gardening can foster a deep sense of connection to the natural world, promoting feelings of peace and tranquility. Similarly, practices like yoga or tai chi, which integrate physical movement with spiritual mindfulness, can enhance both physical and spiritual well-being.

The interconnection between mind, body, and spirit is evident in the concept of **holistic health**, which emphasizes that each component influences and supports the others. For example, managing stress through mindfulness practices can improve mental health, which in turn can lead to better physical health outcomes. Similarly, maintaining physical health through proper nutrition and exercise can enhance mental clarity and emotional stability, while nurturing spiritual health can provide a sense of purpose and fulfillment that supports both mental and physical well-being.

A real-world example of holistic health in practice is the experience of Anna, a woman in her forties who suffered from chronic fatigue and depression. Traditional medical treatments offered little relief, prompting her to explore holistic approaches. Anna adopted a comprehensive wellness plan that included a balanced diet rich in nutrient-dense foods, regular yoga practice, mindfulness meditation, and time spent in nature. Over time, Anna experienced significant improvements in her energy levels, mood, and overall sense of well-being. This transformation underscores the power of integrating mind, body, and spirit in the pursuit of health.

The role of mind, body, and spirit in wellness is central to the holistic health approach. By recognizing and nurturing the interconnections between these elements, individuals can achieve a state of balance and harmony that supports optimal health and well-being. This integrated approach empowers individuals to take an active role in their health, fostering resilience and promoting a fulfilling and vibrant life. As the understanding of holistic health continues to evolve, it offers valuable insights and practices that can enhance the quality of life for individuals and communities alike.

CHAPTER 2
The Power of Nutrition in Natural Healing

2.1 Macronutrients and Micronutrients

In the realm of natural healing, nutrition plays a pivotal role, serving as the foundation upon which the body's health and vitality are built. Understanding the significance of macronutrients and micronutrients is essential for anyone looking to optimize their diet for better health outcomes. These nutrients are the building blocks of life, each playing a unique and vital role in maintaining physiological functions, promoting growth, and preventing disease.

Macronutrients are nutrients that the body requires in relatively large amounts. They include carbohydrates, proteins, and fats, each of which provides energy and contributes to the body's structural and functional integrity.

Carbohydrates are the principal substance that the body uses to generate energy. As a result of their breakdown, glucose is produced, which is then utilized by cells in the production of ATP (adenosine triphosphate), which serves as the energy currency of the cell. The varieties of carbohydrates can be broken down into two categories: basic and complicated. Simple carbs, which can be found in foods such as fruits and honey, are absorbable in a short amount of time and give instant energy. Whole grains, legumes, and vegetables are all sources of complex carbs, which are absorbed more slowly than simple carbohydrates. These carbohydrates provide prolonged energy and contribute to stable blood sugar levels. Consuming a bowl of oats first thing in the morning, for example, is a good example of a slow-release source of energy that can assist in maintaining attention and stamina throughout the afternoon and throughout the day.

Proteins are essential for tissue growth, healing, and maintenance. They contain nine essential amino acids, which must be eaten. Enzymes, hormones, and antibodies, essential for metabolism and immunity, are made from proteins. Protein-rich foods include lean meats, fish, eggs, dairy, legumes, and nuts. Combining protein sources like lentils and quinoa gives a comprehensive amino acid profile for muscle repair and immunological support.

Fats are necessary for a wide variety of body processes, such as the generation of hormones, the formation of cellular structures, and the absorption of fat-soluble vitamins (A, D, E, and K). We can divide fats into three categories: saturated fats, unsaturated fats, and trans fats. Because of their positive effects on cardiovascular health, unsaturated fats, which may be found in foods such as avocados, nuts, seeds, and olive oil, should be given a higher priority in the diet. On the other hand, trans fats, which are frequently present in processed and fried foods, should be reduced as much as possible because of the increased risk of cardiovascular disease that they are associated with. The consumption of omega-3 fatty acids, which are found in fatty fish like salmon, has been demonstrated to assist in the reduction of inflammation and the enhancement of cognitive function.

Micronutrients, on the other hand, are required in smaller quantities but are no less important. These include vitamins and minerals, which are critical for various biochemical processes and overall health maintenance.

Vitamins are chemical substances that play a role in the development of a wide variety of physiological processes. There are two types of vitamins: those that are water-soluble and those that are fat-soluble. Because fat-soluble vitamins (A, D, E, and K) are stored in the fatty tissues and liver of the body, it is not necessary to ingest them on a daily basis that they are consumed. Carrots and sweet potatoes are two examples of foods that contain vitamin A, which is an essential nutrient for maintaining healthy vision and supporting the immune system. It is crucial for bone health and immunological support to consume foods that have been fortified with vitamin D, which is produced by exposure to sunshine and can also be found in fatty fish.

Water-soluble vitamins (B-complex and C) must be consumed regularly as they are not stored in the body. Vitamin C, found in citrus fruits and leafy greens, is important for collagen synthesis, antioxidant protection, and immune function. The B vitamins, found in whole grains, legumes, and animal products, play crucial roles in energy metabolism, red blood cell formation, and neurological function. For instance, a deficiency in vitamin B12, common in strict vegetarians, can lead to anemia and neurological impairments, underscoring the need for dietary or supplementary sources.

Minerals help maintain bone health, fluid balance, and muscle contraction. Large levels of calcium, magnesium, and potassium are needed. Calcium, found in dairy and leafy greens, is essential for bone and muscle health. Nuts, seeds, and whole grains contain magnesium, which is involved in over 300 biochemical activities, including energy synthesis and muscle relaxation.

Although they are required in lesser quantities, trace minerals like iron, zinc, and selenium are just as necessary as their more abundant counterparts. When it comes to oxygen transport in the blood, iron, which can be found in red meat, beans, and spinach, is absolutely necessary. The immune system and the healing of wounds are both supported by zinc, which can be found in nuts, seeds, and meat. The mineral selenium, which may be found in Brazil nuts and seafood, is classified as an antioxidant and is involved in the metabolism of thyroid hormone.

In the context of the prevention of anemia, the value of micronutrients can be seen to be demonstrated for practical purposes. Anemia caused by a lack of iron is a common disorder that can lead to symptoms such as fatigue, weakness, and reduced cognitive function. Individuals are able to prevent this shortage and preserve optimal health by ensuring that they consume a suitable amount of iron-rich foods, such as spinach and lentils, and by improving their iron absorption through the consumption of vitamin C-rich foods, such as oranges and bell peppers.

The interplay between macronutrients and micronutrients is vital for overall health. For instance, the absorption of fat-soluble vitamins is dependent on the presence of dietary fats. A diet that includes healthy fats from sources like avocados and olive oil can enhance the bioavailability of vitamins A, D, E, and K. Similarly, the synthesis of hemoglobin, the oxygen-carrying component of blood, requires both iron and vitamin B6, illustrating the synergistic effects of nutrients.

2.2 Superfoods

The concept of superfoods has gained significant popularity in recent years, celebrated for their dense nutritional profiles and remarkable health benefits. Superfoods are nutrient-rich foods considered particularly beneficial for health and well-being, often containing high levels of vitamins, minerals, antioxidants, and other essential nutrients. They offer a natural and holistic approach to enhancing vitality and preventing disease, fitting seamlessly into the principles of natural healing.

Superfoods are not a new phenomenon; they have been revered for their medicinal and nutritional properties across various cultures for centuries. Their inclusion in the diet can provide an array of health benefits, from boosting the immune system to improving heart health and reducing inflammation.

Blueberries are widely recognized as one of the most powerful superfoods. They are full with antioxidants, particularly anthocyanins, which are responsible for their dark blue hue. These small berries are packed with antioxidants. In order to battle oxidative stress and neutralize free radicals, which are known to cause damage to cells and contribute to the aging process as well as chronic diseases, antioxidants are very necessary. Not only are blueberries abundant in fiber, but they are also abundant in vitamins C and K. Blueberries, when consumed on a regular basis, have been associated with significant improvements in brain function, cardiovascular health, and a decreased chance of developing certain cancers. As an illustration, consuming a serving of blueberries on a daily basis has been shown to enhance memory and cognitive function, making them an advantageous addition to the diet of individuals of all ages.

Another powerful superfood is kale, a dark leafy green vegetable that is incredibly nutrient-dense. Kale is an excellent source of vitamins A, C, and K, as well as folate, manganese, and calcium. Its high fiber content aids digestion and supports a healthy gut microbiome. The presence of antioxidants like quercetin and kaempferol helps reduce inflammation and protect against chronic diseases. Consuming kale in salads, smoothies, or as a sautéed side dish can significantly boost one's nutritional intake.

- **Chia seeds:** are yet another outstanding superfood that are well-known for their high levels of omega-3 fatty acids, fiber, protein, and vital minerals such as calcium and magnesium. The health of the heart, the reduction of inflammation, and the support of brain function are all critically dependent on omega-3 fatty acids. Because they take on a gel-like consistency when they are soaked in liquid, chia seeds are a fantastic addition to puddings, smoothies, and yogurt. They provide prolonged energy and promote satiety, making them an excellent choice for these beverages.
- **Salmon:** especially wild-caught types, is treasured for its high omega-3 fatty acid content, especially EPA and DHA, which enhance cardiovascular health, inflammation reduction, and cognitive function. Salmon is rich in omega-3s, protein, B vitamins, and selenium. Salmon eating reduces heart disease risk, improves mental wellness, and strengthens joints. Grilled or baked salmon is a healthy main entrée.
- **Avocados:** another heart-healthy superfood with monounsaturated fats. Fiber, potassium, vitamins E, C, and B-6 are abundant. Avocados' potassium regu-

lates blood pressure and their beneficial fats lower cholesterol and inflammation. Avocados provide flavor and versatility to salads, sandwiches, smoothies, and guacamole.

- **Turmeric:** a golden-yellow spice commonly used in Indian cuisine, is celebrated for its powerful anti-inflammatory and antioxidant properties. The active compound in turmeric, curcumin, has been extensively studied for its potential health benefits, including reducing inflammation, combating oxidative stress, and improving brain health. Turmeric can be added to curries, teas, and smoothies, or taken as a supplement to harness its therapeutic properties. For example, a daily dose of turmeric can help alleviate symptoms of arthritis and improve overall joint health.
- **Quinoa:** a gluten-free grain, is considered a superfood due to its high protein content and balanced amino acid profile. It is also rich in fiber, magnesium, B vitamins, and iron. Quinoa's versatility makes it an excellent substitute for rice or pasta, and it can be used in salads, soups, and as a side dish. Its high protein and fiber content make it particularly beneficial for vegetarians and those looking to increase their protein intake without relying on animal products.
- **Dark chocolate:** with a high cocoa content (70% or higher) is another superfood worth mentioning. Rich in antioxidants, particularly flavonoids, dark chocolate has been shown to improve heart health, enhance brain function, and reduce inflammation. Moderate consumption of dark chocolate can lower blood pressure, improve blood flow, and protect the skin from sun damage. Enjoying a small piece of dark chocolate daily can satisfy sweet cravings while providing significant health benefits.
- **Garlic:** is a superfood known for its potent medicinal properties. Rich in sulfur compounds like allicin, garlic has been shown to boost the immune system, reduce blood pressure, and improve cholesterol levels. It also has antimicrobial and antiviral properties, making it a valuable food for preventing infections and supporting overall health. Incorporating garlic into daily meals, such as in sauces, dressings, and roasted vegetables, can enhance flavor and provide health benefits.

It is possible that the addition of superfoods to one's diet can have a significant impact on one's health and well-being. The natural healing processes of the body are supported by these nutrient-dense foods, which give the body with important vitamins, minerals, antioxidants, and healthy fats. It is possible for individuals to improve their nutritional intake, strengthen their immune system, reduce inflammation, and protect themselves against chronic diseases by incorporating a range of superfoods into their daily nutritional intake.

For instance, a typical day incorporating superfoods might start with a smoothie made from kale, blueberries, chia seeds, and almond milk. Lunch could include a quinoa salad with avocado, tomatoes, and a lemon-turmeric dressing. Dinner might feature grilled salmon with a side of garlic-roasted vegetables. For dessert, a small piece of dark chocolate can satisfy a sweet tooth while providing antioxidant benefits.

2.3 Detoxification

Detoxification is a fundamental concept in natural healing, emphasizing the body's ability to cleanse itself of toxins and restore optimal function. The process of detoxification involves the elimination of harmful substances from the body, which can accumulate due to environmental pollutants, poor dietary choices, and metabolic by-products. By understanding the mechanisms of detoxification and employing natural strategies to support this vital process, individuals can enhance their overall health and well-being.

The human body is equipped with a sophisticated detoxification system that primarily involves the liver, kidneys, intestines, lungs, skin, and lymphatic system. Each of these organs plays a specific role in identifying, neutralizing, and eliminating toxins. The liver, for instance, is the body's primary detoxification organ, performing complex biochemical reactions to convert fat-soluble toxins into water-soluble compounds that can be excreted via urine or bile.

In the liver, detoxification occurs in two phases:

- **Phase I detoxification:** involves the use of enzymes, particularly the cytochrome P450 family, to modify toxins through oxidation, reduction, or hydrolysis. These reactions often produce reactive intermediates that can be more harmful than the original toxins.
- **Phase II detoxification:** involves conjugation reactions, where molecules such as glutathione, sulfate, or glycine are attached to the toxins, making them water-soluble and easier to excrete. Supporting both phases of liver detoxification is crucial for effective toxin elimination.

By filtering the blood, the kidneys eliminate waste products and compounds that are in excess, and they then excrete these items in the urine. Consuming an adequate amount of water is necessary in order to maintain healthy kidney function and guarantee the effective removal of water-soluble pollutants. Maintaining kidney health and promoting detoxification can be accomplished by consuming a large amount of water and herbal teas, such as those made from dandelion or nettle flower.

The gut detoxifies too. The gut microbiota breaks down toxins and produces short-chain fatty acids for intestinal health. Fiber-rich fruits, vegetables, and whole grains stimulate regular bowel movements, which help eliminate pollutants. Fermented foods like yogurt, kefir, and sauerkraut include probiotics that aid digestion and detoxification.

The lungs expel volatile toxins and metabolic by-products through exhalation. Practices such as deep breathing, yoga, and aerobic exercise can improve lung capacity and efficiency, enhancing the elimination of gaseous toxins. Additionally, spending time in environments with clean, fresh air can reduce the burden on the respiratory system and support overall detoxification.

The skin is the body's largest organ and acts as a barrier to external toxins while also participating in detoxification through sweating. Regular physical activity that induces sweating, such as exercise or using a sauna, can help eliminate toxins through the skin. Skin brushing and the use of natural exfoliants can further support detoxification by removing dead skin cells and promoting circulation.

The lymphatic system, comprising a network of lymph nodes and vessels, transports lymph fluid throughout the body to collect and remove waste products, pathogens, and toxins. Unlike the circulatory system, the lymphatic system does not have a central pump and relies on muscle contractions to move lymph fluid. Regular exercise, massage, and practices such as dry brushing can stimulate lymphatic flow and enhance detoxification.

In addition to supporting the body's natural detoxification pathways, certain dietary and lifestyle practices can further aid in the elimination of toxins:

When it comes to detoxifying, **dietary**

choices are of the utmost importance. In order to neutralize free radicals and prevent oxidative stress, it is possible to consume a diet that is abundant in antioxidants, which may be found in colorful fruits and vegetables. Sulforaphane is one of the substances found in cruciferous vegetables including broccoli, cauliflower, and Brussels sprouts. These foods contain components that boost the enzymes that are responsible for liver detoxification in Phase II.

Herbal remedies can also support detoxification:

- **Milk thistle (Silybum marianum):** is well-known for its hepatoprotective properties, promoting liver health and enhancing detoxification.
- **Dandelion root (Taraxacum officinale):** acts as a diuretic, supporting kidney function and the elimination of toxins through urine.
- **Burdock root (Arctium lappa):** is another herb that supports liver detoxification and promotes healthy skin.

Intermittent fasting and juice cleanses are popular detoxification strategies that give the digestive system a break, allowing the body to focus on eliminating toxins:

- **Intermittent fasting:** a cellular process that eliminates damaged components and promotes cellular renewal is called autophagy. Intermittent fasting comprises periods of reduced food consumption, which can trigger autophagy.

- **Juice cleanses:** typically involve consuming only fruit and vegetable juices for a set period, providing a concentrated source of vitamins, minerals, and antioxidants while reducing the burden on the digestive system.

A real-world example of the benefits of detoxification can be seen in individuals who undertake a structured detox program. For instance, Sarah, a woman in her late thirties, struggled with chronic fatigue, digestive issues, and frequent headaches. After consulting with a naturopath, she embarked on a two-week detox program that included a diet of whole, organic foods, plenty of water, and specific herbal supplements like milk thistle and dandelion root. She also incorporated daily exercise, deep breathing exercises, and sauna sessions. By the end of the program, Sarah reported increased energy levels, improved digestion, and a significant reduction in headaches, demonstrating the effectiveness of a comprehensive detoxification approach.

Detoxification is a critical component of natural healing that involves the removal of toxins from the body to restore and maintain health. By supporting the liver, kidneys, intestines, lungs, skin, and lymphatic system through proper nutrition, hydration, exercise, and the use of herbal remedies, individuals can enhance their body's natural ability to detoxify. Embracing detoxification practices as part of a holistic health regimen can lead to improved vitality, resilience, and overall well-being.

CHAPTER 3
Herbs and Their Uses

3.1 Introduction to Herbal Medicine

Herbal medicine, one of the oldest forms of healthcare, harnesses the therapeutic properties of plants to prevent and treat a wide range of ailments. This practice dates back thousands of years, with evidence of its use in ancient civilizations such as Egypt, China, and India. Herbal medicine is not just a relic of the past; it continues to be an integral part of modern healthcare, offering natural and effective remedies that complement conventional treatments. Understanding the foundations of herbal medicine involves exploring its historical roots, the principles guiding its use, and its applications in contemporary wellness practices.

On the basis of the utilization of medicinal plants and plant extracts, herbal medicine, which is sometimes referred to as phytotherapy, is practiced. Alkaloids, flavonoids, tannins, and glycosides are just some of the bioactive substances that can be found in these plants. These compounds have the potential to have therapeutic effects on the body at various levels. Herbal treatments, on the other hand, often have a holistic effect, which means that they support overall health and enhance the body's natural healing processes. This is in contrast to synthetic pharmaceuticals, which frequently target specific symptoms or biochemical pathways.

The history of herbal medicine is rich and varied, reflecting the diverse cultures that have contributed to its development. In Ancient Egypt, the Ebers Papyrus, dating back to 1550 BCE, documents the use of over 700 plant-based remedies. This ancient text highlights the Egyptians' advanced understanding of herbal medicine, which they used to treat ailments ranging from digestive disorders to infections.

Herbal remedies have balanced qi for over 3,000 years in Traditional Chinese Medicine (TCM). TCM stresses balance between body systems and nature. Complex TCM herbal formulae address imbalances and improve health by combining numerous plants. Ginseng (Panax ginseng) is known for its adaptogenic effects, which boost energy and stress resilience.

Herbal medicine is also given a large amount of importance in Ayurveda, which is an ancient medical system that originated in India. Practitioners of Ayurveda make use of herbs in order to bring the body's three doshas—vata, pitta, and kapha—into harmony. These doshas are considered to be responsible for the body's physical and mental activities. Turmeric, also known as Curcuma longa, is a staple in Ayurvedic medicine. It is used to treat a wide range of diseases, including arthritis and skin disorders, due to its anti-inflammatory and antioxidant characteristics.

In Western herbal medicine, which has evolved from the traditions of Ancient Greece and Rome, the use of herbs is guided by principles such as the "doctrine of signatures." This principle suggests that the physical characteristics of a plant indicate its therapeutic uses. For example, the bright red berries of hawthorn (Crataegus spp.) are associated with heart health, and hawthorn has indeed been used traditionally to support cardiovascular function.

One of the key advantages of herbal medicine is its holistic approach to health. Herbs are often used to support the body's natural defenses and improve overall wellness rather than just treating specific symptoms. This approach can lead to more sustainable health outcomes, as it addresses the underlying causes of illness and promotes long-term balance.

Echinacea (Echinacea purpurea) is used to enhance immunity and prevent colds and flu. Echinacea has been demonstrated to boost macrophage and natural killer cell activity, helping the body fight infections. Echinacea boosts immunity and promotes health and resilience.

Similarly, milk thistle (Silybum marianum) is a well-known herb for liver health. Its active compound, silymarin, has been shown to protect liver cells from toxins, reduce inflammation, and support liver regeneration. This makes milk thistle an excellent choice for individuals seeking to detoxify their bodies and support liver function.

There are also treatments available for reducing stress and improving mental well-being that can be found in herbal medicine. Adaptogenic herbs, which include ashwagandha (Withania somnifera) and rhodiola (Rhodiola rosea), assist the body in adjusting to stress and mitigate the adverse effects that prolonged stress can have on one's health. For instance, ashwagandha has been demonstrated to reduce levels of the stress hormone cortisol, improve mood, and promote cognitive performance. As a result, it is an extreme-ly useful herb for improving mental and emotional equilibrium for individuals.

The versatility of herbal medicine is evident in its application across various health conditions. For digestive health, herbs like ginger (Zingiber officinale) and peppermint (Mentha piperita) can provide relief from nausea, bloating, and indigestion. Ginger's anti-inflammatory properties and ability to stimulate digestion make it a popular remedy for gastrointestinal discomfort, while peppermint's antispasmodic effects can help to relax the muscles of the digestive tract and alleviate symptoms of irritable bowel syndrome (IBS).

In skincare, herbs like calendula (Calendula officinalis) and aloe vera (Aloe barbadensis) are prized for their soothing and healing properties. Calendula's anti-inflammatory and antimicrobial effects make it an excellent choice for treating wounds, burns, and skin irritations, while aloe vera's moisturizing and healing properties are beneficial for soothing sunburns and promoting skin health.

Herbal medicine uses concentrated plant extracts called essential oils. Lavender and tea tree essential oils are powerful therapeutic agents that can be utilized in aromatherapy, topical treatments, and natural cleaning. Lavender essential oil is popular for calming and relaxing, encouraging sleep and lowering anxiety. With its antibacterial and anti-inflammatory characteristics, tea tree oil is extensively used to treat acne, fungal infections, and minor wounds.

A practical example of herbal medicine in action can be seen in the treatment of common colds. When someone feels the onset of a cold, they might prepare a tea made from elderberries (Sambucus nigra) and echinacea. Elderberries are rich in antioxidants and have been shown to reduce the severity and duration of cold symptoms. Combining elderberries with echinacea can enhance the immune-boosting effects, helping to ward off the cold more quickly.

3.2 Growing, Harvesting, and Storing Herbs

The practice of growing, harvesting, and storing herbs is an essential aspect of herbal medicine, ensuring a sustainable and consistent supply of high-quality medicinal plants. Cultivating your own herbs not only provides access to fresh and potent ingredients but also fosters a deeper connection to the natural world and the healing properties of plants. This comprehensive approach involves understanding the specific needs of different herbs, the best practices for harvesting, and the methods for preserving their therapeutic qualities.

Growing herbs begins with selecting the appropriate species for your climate and growing conditions. Herbs can be grown in a variety of settings, from large outdoor gardens to small indoor pots, making them accessible to both rural and urban dwellers. Key factors to consider include sunlight, soil quality, water requirements, and space.

- **Sunlight:** Most herbs require full sunlight, meaning at least six hours of direct sunlight per day. Herbs like rosemary, thyme, and sage thrive in sunny locations, while others, such as mint and parsley, can tolerate partial shade.
- **Soil Quality:** Healthy herb growth requires well-draining soil. Many herbs like soil pH 6.0–7.5. Organic stuff like compost or old manure improves soil fertility and structure.
- **Water Requirements:** Herbs generally prefer consistent moisture but should not be waterlogged. Overwatering can lead to root rot and other fungal diseases. It's important to understand the specific water needs of each herb; for example, Mediterranean herbs like lavender and oregano prefer drier conditions, while basil and cilantro require more frequent watering.
- **Space:** Consider the mature size of the herb plants when planning your garden layout. Some herbs, such as mint, can be invasive and should be planted in containers to prevent them from overtaking other plants.

Once the herbs are established and thriving, the next step is harvesting. The timing and method of harvesting can significantly impact the potency and efficacy of the herbs.

- **Timing:** The best time to harvest herbs is typically in the morning after the dew has dried but before the heat of the day. This ensures that the plants are not stressed by heat and retain their essential oils, which are often at their peak in the morning. For most herbs, harvesting just before they flower provides the highest concentration of active compounds.
- **Method:** Use sharp scissors or pruning shears to cut the herbs, ensuring a clean cut that minimizes damage to the plant. For leafy herbs like basil and mint, pinch or cut the stems just above a leaf node to encourage bushier growth. For herbs like rosemary and thyme, which grow on woody stems, take cuttings from the soft, new growth.

Proper storage is essential to maintain the potency and quality of harvested herbs. There are several methods for preserving herbs, depending on their intended use and the available resources.

Drying Herbs:
- **Air Drying:** This is one of the simplest and most effective methods for drying herbs. Bundle small bunches of herbs together and hang them upside down in a warm, dry, and well-ventilated area,

away from direct sunlight. Air drying is suitable for herbs with low moisture content, such as rosemary, thyme, and oregano.

- **Dehydrating:** Using a food dehydrator allows for controlled drying conditions and is especially useful for herbs with higher moisture content, like basil and parsley. Set the dehydrator to a low temperature (95-115°F or 35-46°C) to preserve the herbs' color, flavor, and medicinal properties.

Freezing Herbs:

- **Whole Leaves:** For herbs like basil, cilantro, and parsley, freezing can preserve their fresh flavor. Rinse and dry the leaves thoroughly, then spread them on a baking sheet and freeze until solid. Transfer the frozen leaves to an airtight container or freezer bag.
- **Herb Cubes:** Chop herbs and set them in ice cube trays with water or olive oil. Transfer herb cubes from frozen trays to freezer bags for easy portioning in soups, stews, and sauces.

Infusing in Oil or Vinegar:

- **Herbal Oils:** Herbal oil infusions provide strong culinary and medicinal extracts. Fill a clean, dry jar with fresh or dried herbs and cover with high-quality olive or coconut oil. Seal the jar and shake it occasionally in a warm, bright position for many weeks. Use a fine mesh screen or cheesecloth to strain the oil.
- **Herbal Vinegars:** Are prepared by steeping herbs in vinegar, like oil infusions. The basis should be apple cider or white wine vinegar. Pour vinegar over herbs in a container and let sit for weeks, shaking occasionally. Strain and bottle vinegar for dressings, marinades, and tonics.

Storing Dried Herbs:

- **Airtight Containers:** To maintain the effectiveness of dried herbs, store them in airtight jars away from heat, light, and moisture. The best glass jars have tight-fitting lids. For the purpose of monitoring freshness, mark the containers with the name of the plant and the harvest date.
- **Vacuum Sealing:** For longer-term storage, consider vacuum-sealing dried herbs to remove air and prevent oxidation. This method can extend the shelf life of dried herbs for up to two years.

A practical example of these principles in action is the cultivation and use of lavender (Lavandula angustifolia). Lavender thrives in well-draining soil and full sun, making it ideal for Mediterranean climates. Harvest lavender just as the flowers begin to open, when their essential oil content is highest. Cut the flower spikes and bundle them for air drying in a dark, dry space. Once dried, lavender can be stored in airtight containers or used to make herbal sachets, infused oils, or calming teas.

In conclusion, growing, harvesting, and storing herbs require careful attention to the needs of each plant and the conditions in which they thrive. By following best practices for cultivation and preservation, individuals can ensure a steady supply of high-quality herbs for culinary, medicinal, and therapeutic use. This process not only enhances the potency and efficacy of herbal remedies but also fosters a deeper appreciation for the natural world and its healing potential.

3.3 Setting Up Your Home Apothecary

Establishing a home apothecary is an enriching endeavor that brings the ancient art of herbal medicine into your everyday life. A well-organized home apothecary allows you to create, store, and use herbal remedies tailored to your health needs, fostering self-reliance and a deeper connection to natural healing. Setting up a home apothecary involves selecting essential tools and supplies, organizing your workspace, and ensuring proper storage to maintain the potency and effectiveness of your herbal preparations.

The first step in setting up your home apothecary is to gather the necessary tools and supplies. These items are fundamental for preparing and storing herbal remedies:

- **Mortar and Pestle:** Essential for grinding herbs into powders or pastes. This traditional tool is excellent for breaking down tough plant materials and releasing their active compounds.
- **Herb Grinder:** For more efficient and consistent grinding of dried herbs, an electric herb grinder can be very useful, especially when dealing with larger quantities.
- **Mixing Bowls and Spoons:** Various sizes of mixing bowls and non-reactive spoons (wooden or stainless steel) are needed for blending herbs and making tinctures, salves, and teas.
- **Strainers and Cheesecloth:** Fine mesh strainers and cheesecloth are essential for filtering out plant material from liquid preparations like infusions, decoctions, and tinctures.
- **Glass Jars and Bottles:** Airtight glass jars and bottles in various sizes are crucial for storing dried herbs, tinctures, infused oils, and other preparations. Dark amber or cobalt blue bottles help protect contents from light degradation.
- **Measuring Tools:** Accurate measurements are critical in herbal medicine. Include a set of measuring spoons, cups, and a digital scale for precise dosing.
- **Labels and Markers:** Proper labeling

of all preparations is essential. Labels should include the herb name, preparation date, and any specific instructions or expiration dates.
- **Double Boiler:** Useful for making salves and balms, a double boiler ensures gentle, even heating to prevent burning delicate herbs and oils.

Creating a dedicated space for your home apothecary helps keep your herbal practice organized and efficient. This space can be as simple as a kitchen cabinet or as elaborate as a dedicated room, depending on your needs and available space. Consider the following tips for organizing your apothecary:

- **Shelving and Storage:** Install sturdy shelves to store jars and bottles. Ensure that the shelves are easily accessible and strong enough to hold the weight of glass containers filled with herbs and liquids.
- **Workspace:** A clean, flat workspace, such as a countertop or table, is necessary for preparing and mixing herbs. Make sure this area is well-lit and free from contaminants.
- **Storage Containers:** Use airtight glass jars for storing dried herbs to maintain their potency. Mason jars are a popular choice, and labeling each jar with the herb name and date of harvest ensures proper identification and freshness.
- **Drawers and Bins:** Drawers or bins can be used to store smaller tools and supplies like strainers, cheesecloth, and measuring spoons, keeping them organized and within easy reach.
- **Refrigeration:** Some preparations, like certain tinctures and infused oils, may require refrigeration to extend their shelf life. Allocate space in your refrigerator for these items.

Proper storage is crucial to maintain the efficacy of your herbal remedies. Herbs and herbal preparations are susceptible to degradation from light, heat, and moisture. Here are some key storage practices:

- **Light Protection:** Store herbs and herbal preparations in dark glass containers to protect them from light exposure, which can degrade their active compounds. Keep these containers in a dark cabinet or pantry.
- **Temperature Control:** Store herbs in a cool, dry place to prevent the growth of mold and the breakdown of active ingredients. Avoid areas near heat sources like stoves or direct sunlight.
- **Moisture Control:** Moisture can cause dried herbs to mold. Use desiccants, such as silica gel packets, in storage containers to absorb excess moisture. Ensure jars and bottles are sealed tightly to keep out humidity.
- **Rotation and Inventory:** Practice the principle of "first in, first out" (FIFO) to ensure you use the oldest preparations first, maintaining the freshness of your stock. Regularly check your inventory and replenish supplies as needed.
- **Documentation:** Keep detailed records of your herbal preparations, including recipes, dates of preparation, and any observations. This practice helps track the efficacy of your remedies and refine your formulations over time.

Practical Example: Creating and Storing a Calendula Salve

Let's illustrate the process with a practical example: making and storing a calendula (Calendula officinalis) salve, renowned for its skin-soothing properties.

Gather Ingredients and Tools:

- Dried calendula flowers
- Olive oil
- Beeswax
- Double boiler
- Strainer or cheesecloth
- Mixing bowls
- Glass jars for storage

Fill a clean jar with dried calendula flowers. Pour olive oil over the flowers, making sure they are well submerged. For 2-4 weeks, keep the jar sealed and place it in a warm, sunny position. Shake the jar often to aid in the infusion process. Alternatively, to expedite the process, gradually heat the oil and flowers for many hours using a double boiler.

Once the infusion period has ended, the plant debris should be removed from the oil by straining it through cheesecloth or a strainer with fine mesh. Using a clean and dry container, pour the oil that has been filtered. Using a measuring cup, pour the oil that has been infused into the top of a double boiler. To the oil, add beeswax at a ratio of approximately one ounce of beeswax to every four ounces of oil. Allow the beeswax to melt completely while stirring it occasionally while it is being heated softly. Take the mixture off the stove and pour it into small glass jars or tins while it is still warm and liquid. Each jar should be labeled with the contents as well as the date.

Allow the salve to cool and solidify before sealing the jars. Store the jars in a cool, dark place to maintain the salve's potency.

By setting up a well-organized home apothecary, you can ensure a steady supply of high-quality herbal remedies tailored to your needs. This practice not only supports your health but also deepens your connection to the natural world and the time-honored traditions of herbal medicine.

CHAPTER 4
Key Herbs for Natural Healing

4.1 Chamomile: The Calming Healer

Chamomile (Matricaria chamomilla), often referred to as the "calming healer," is a beloved herb in the realm of natural healing, renowned for its soothing and therapeutic properties. This unassuming plant, with its daisy-like flowers and sweet, apple-like scent, has been used for centuries in various cultures to treat a wide array of ailments. Chamomile's gentle yet effective actions make it a staple in herbal medicine, particularly valued for its calming, anti-inflammatory, and digestive benefits.

Chamomile's reputation as a calming agent is perhaps its most well-known attribute. The herb contains several bioactive compounds, including flavonoids and terpenoids, which contribute to its sedative and anxiolytic effects. Apigenin, a flavonoid found in chamomile, binds to benzodiazepine receptors in the brain, promoting relaxation and reducing anxiety without the side effects associated with pharmaceutical sedatives. Drinking chamomile tea before bedtime is a common practice for those seeking to improve sleep quality and alleviate insomnia. The gentle sedative properties of chamomile help to ease tension and prepare the body and mind for restful sleep.

In addition to its relaxing benefits, chamomile is also an effective anti-inflammatory drug. It is primarily owing to the presence of alpha-bisabolol and matricin, which are chemicals that suppress the formation of inflammatory mediators, that the herb possesses anti-inflammatory qualities. Because of this, chamomile is a useful treatment for illnesses that are characterized by inflammation, such as arthritis, muscle discomfort, and disorders of the gastrointestinal tract. Consuming chamomile in the form of a tea or using it topically in the form of a compress or ointment will accomplish the same goals of reducing inflammation and soothing sensitive areas.

Chamomile's benefits extend to digestive health as well. The herb has been traditionally used to treat various digestive complaints, including indigestion, bloating, gas, and colic. Chamomile's antispasmodic properties help to relax the smooth muscles of the digestive tract, alleviating spasms and cramps. Additionally, its mild bitter principles stimulate the production of digestive enzymes and bile, enhancing overall digestion. For individuals suffering from irritable bowel syndrome (IBS) or other gastrointestinal disturbances, chamomile tea can provide significant relief and promote a more comfortable digestive process.

Chamomile's versatility as a healing herb is further demonstrated by its application in skincare. The herb's anti-inflammatory, antimicrobial, and antioxidant properties make it an excellent choice for treating various skin conditions, such as eczema, dermatitis, and minor wounds. Chamomile-infused oils, creams, and lotions can be applied to the skin to reduce redness, irritation, and inflammation. For example, a chamomile compress made by soaking a clean cloth in chamomile tea and applying it to the affected area can soothe sunburns, rashes, and insect bites.

A practical example of chamomile's efficacy is its use in managing childhood ailments. Chamomile is gentle enough for use with infants and children, making it a popular remedy for teething pain, colic, and irritability. A warm chamomile tea bath can help calm a fussy baby and promote better sleep. Additionally, a few drops of chamomile tincture diluted in water can be given to alleviate colic and digestive discomfort in infants.

Chamomile's role in natural healing is supported by modern scientific research, which continues to uncover the herb's broad range of therapeutic effects. Studies have shown that chamomile's anti-inflammatory and antioxidant properties may also contribute to its potential in cancer prevention and treatment. The herb's ability to induce apoptosis (programmed cell death) in cancer cells, without harming healthy cells, highlights its potential as a complementary therapy in oncology.

Chamomile is easy to prepare and use at home. Put one to two tablespoons of dried chamomile flowers in a cup of hot water for 5-10 minutes to prepare tea. Strain and drink the tea three times a day for digestion and tranquility. Chamomile can be steeped in olive or almond oil and applied to the skin or added to bathwater for a calming soak.

4.2 Echinacea: Immune System Booster

Echinacea (Echinacea purpurea), commonly known as the purple coneflower, is a powerful herb widely recognized for its immune-boosting properties. Originating from North America, echinacea has been used by Indigenous peoples for centuries to treat infections and wounds. Today, it remains a popular natural remedy for enhancing immune function and combating various infections, particularly those of the upper respiratory tract.

The rich composition of bioactive chemicals found in echinacea, which includes alkamides, glycoproteins, polysaccharides, and caffeic acid derivatives like echinacoside and chicoric acid, is responsible for the immune-enhancing properties of this plant. White blood cells are essential for the fight against infections, and these substances work together to stimulate the immune system in a way that is synergistic, so increasing the generation of white blood cells and their activity.

One of the key ways in which echinacea improves immune function is by promoting phagocytosis. Phagocytosis is the process by which immune cells, such as macrophages, consume and eliminate invaders like bacteria and viruses. In addition, echinacea stimulates the creation of interferons, which are proteins that are essential to the body's defense mechanism against viral infections. Due to this, echinacea is particularly helpful in lowering the severity of colds and flu as well as the duration of their symptoms.

Several studies have demonstrated echinacea's effectiveness in boosting immune response. A meta-analysis of clinical trials found that echinacea can reduce the risk of developing the common cold by 58% and shorten the duration of colds by 1.4 days. These findings support the traditional use of echinacea as a preventive measure during cold and flu season.

In addition to its immune-stimulating properties, echinacea possesses anti-inflammatory effects. The herb's alkamides and caffeic acid derivatives inhibit the production of pro-inflammatory cytokines, which are involved in the inflammatory response. This makes echinacea beneficial for managing inflammatory conditions such as bronchitis and sinusitis, where inflammation plays a significant role in symptom severity.

Echinacea is also noted for its antiviral and antimicrobial properties. The herb has been shown to inhibit the replication of various viruses, including influenza and herpes simplex viruses. Its antimicrobial effects extend to bacteria and fungi, making echinacea a versatile remedy for a wide range of infections. For example, echinacea can be used as a supportive treatment for urinary tract infections (UTIs) and skin infections.

The use of echinacea in the early stages of an upper respiratory infection is one example of a practical application of this medication. By taking echinacea at the first sign of symptoms, such as a sore throat or runny nose, one can help strengthen the immune system and prevent the illness from going further. Teas, tinctures, capsules, and extracts are just some of the ways that echinacea can be eaten that are available to consumers. When treating acute infections, it is frequently advisable to take a greater dosage on a more frequent basis during the beginning of the symptoms.

Echinacea tea is easy to make and boosts immunity. Steep one to two tablespoons of dried echinacea root or aerial parts in boiling water for 10-15 minutes to prepare tea. Drink the tea three times a day after straining. Echinacea's immune-boosting qualities are harnessed gently but effectively.

For a more concentrated form, echinacea tinctures are a convenient option. Tinctures are alcohol-based extracts that preserve the active compounds of the herb, providing a potent and easily absorbed form of echinacea. To use a tincture, follow the manufacturer's dosage instructions, typically around 1-2 ml taken up to three times daily at the first sign of illness.

Echinacea can also be combined with other immune-boosting herbs for enhanced effect. For instance, combining echinacea with elderberry (Sambucus nigra) creates a powerful remedy for viral infections. Elderberry is rich in antioxidants and has been shown to inhibit the replication of influenza viruses, making it an excellent complementary herb to echinacea.

It is crucial to highlight that those who have allergies to plants belonging to the Asteraceae family (such as ragweed, chrysanthemums, marigolds, and daisies) should use echinacea with caution. Although echinacea is typically safe for most people, it is vital to remember that this classification is not universally applicable. Furthermore, individuals who are living with autoimmune disorders or who are on immunosuppressive treatments should seek the advice of a medical professional prior to using echinacea. This is because the immune-stimulating effects of echinacea may interact with the therapy or condition that they are currently experiencing.

4.3 Ginger: Digestive Aid and Anti-Inflammatory

Ginger (Zingiber officinale) is a widely celebrated herb known for its powerful digestive and anti-inflammatory properties. This aromatic rhizome has been used for thousands of years in traditional medicine systems across the globe, including Ayurveda, Traditional Chinese Medicine, and ancient Greek medicine. Its versatility and effectiveness make it a staple in natural healing practices, particularly for addressing digestive issues and reducing inflammation.

The capacity of ginger to increase the synthesis of digestive enzymes and bile, which in turn improves the digestive process as a whole, is the primary reason for the digestive benefits that ginger provides. Ginger is a good therapy for a variety of gastrointestinal disorders, including indigestion, bloating, and gas, as a result of this property. It has been demonstrated that the active chemicals found in ginger, such as gingerols and shogaols, facilitate the flow of food through the digestive tract, thereby alleviating the symptoms of indigestion and enhancing the body's ability to absorb nutrients.

One of the most common uses of ginger is to alleviate nausea and vomiting. Ginger has proven particularly effective in managing nausea related to pregnancy (morning sickness), motion sickness, and postoperative recovery. For example, a study published in the "Journal of Obstetrics and Gynaecology" found that ginger significantly reduced the severity of nausea and vomiting in pregnant women. Similarly, another study demonstrated that ginger was as effective as conventional anti-nausea medications in preventing motion sickness.

Similarly impressive are the anti-inflammatory qualities that ginger possesses. Chronic inflammation is a fundamental factor in the development of a wide range of disorders, including metabolic syndrome, cardiovascular diseases, and arthritis. Ginger's capacity to block the production of pro-inflammatory cytokines and enzymes, such as cyclooxygenase (COX) and lipoxygenase (LOX), is the primary reason for its anti-inflammatory results. Ginger has been shown to have anti-inflammatory properties. Because of this activity, ginger is an effective natural medicine for illnesses such as osteoarthritis and rheumatoid arthritis. It helps reduce inflammation and pain.

For instance, a study published in "Arthritis & Rheumatism" showed that patients with osteoarthritis of the knee who consumed ginger experienced significant reductions in pain and improvements in physical function compared to those who took a placebo. This makes ginger a compelling option for individuals seeking natural alternatives to nonsteroidal anti-inflammatory drugs (NSAIDs), which can have adverse side effects with long-term use.

Ginger protects cells from free radical damage with its antioxidant qualities. Oxidative stress from free radicals damages cells and causes chronic illnesses. Gingerols and zingerone neutralize free radicals and minimize oxidative stress, improving health.

A practical example of ginger's effectiveness can be seen in its use for treating cold and flu symptoms. Ginger's warming properties help to stimulate circulation and promote sweating, which can aid in breaking a fever and expelling toxins from the body. Additionally, its antiviral and antibacterial properties help combat the pathogens that cause colds and flu. Drinking ginger tea is a common remedy for soothing sore throats, reducing congestion, and providing relief from the chills and aches associated with these illnesses.

To prepare ginger tea, simply slice a fresh piece of ginger root (about 1-2 inches) and steep it in boiling water for 10-15 minutes. Adding a squeeze of lemon and a teaspoon of honey not only enhances the flavor but also boosts the tea's immune-supporting properties. Drinking this tea 2-3 times a day can help alleviate symptoms and support recovery from colds and flu.

In addition to teas, ginger can be incorporated into the diet in various forms, including fresh, dried, powdered, and as an extract or oil. Fresh ginger can be added to smoothies, soups, and stir-fries to enhance flavor and provide digestive benefits. Dried or powdered ginger is commonly used in baking and cooking, offering a convenient way to include ginger's health benefits in everyday meals.

Ginger's versatility extends to topical applications as well. Ginger oil, when diluted with a carrier oil such as coconut or olive oil, can be used for massage to relieve muscle pain and joint stiffness. The warming sensation of ginger oil helps improve blood circulation and reduce inflammation in the affected areas. Additionally, ginger compresses, made by soaking a cloth in warm ginger tea and applying it to sore muscles or joints, can provide targeted relief from pain and inflammation.

It is essential to use ginger in moderation and to be aware of the potential interactions that it may have with certain medications, despite the fact that ginger is generally safe for the majority of individuals. Ginger, for example, has the potential to improve the effects of anticoagulant drugs, which in turn can increase the risk of becoming bleeding. Consequently, persons who are currently using blood thinners or any other medications should seek the advice of a healthcare expert prior to utilizing ginger as a treatment.

4.4 Lavender: Stress Reliever and Sleep Aid

The **lavender** plant, also known as **Lavandula angustifolia**, is a well-liked herb that is well-known for its calming and relaxing effects. As a result, it is a popular choice for its ability to alleviate stress and improve sleep. Since ancient times, its fragrant purple blooms have been utilized in a variety of purposes, including aromatherapy, traditional medicine, and even culinary applications. Essential oils derived from lavender contain a wide range of bioactive chemicals, including linalool and linalyl acetate, which are responsible for the therapeutic advantages of lavender. It has been demonstrated via comprehensive research and validation that these chemicals have the capacity to increase the quality of sleep, as well as to promote relaxation and reduce anxiety.

The use of lavender as a natural cure for stress and anxiety is one of the most common applications of this plant. Both the mind and the body can benefit from the calming effects of lavender's aroma, which has a direct influence on the neurological system when inhaled. The inhalation of lavender essential oil has the potential to lower levels of cortisol, which is the principal stress hormone in the body, so significantly lowering the total stress response. For instance, a study that was published in the "Journal of Alternative and Complementary Medicine" discovered that participants who inhaled lavender essential oil prior to undertaking a stressful activity experienced considerably lower levels of anxiety and increased mood in comparison to those who did not inhale the oil.

Lavender's anxiolytic effects can also be harnessed through various forms of aromatherapy. Diffusing lavender essential oil in a room can create a tranquil atmosphere, ideal for relaxation and unwinding after a long day. Additionally, lavender sachets placed under pillows or in closets can provide a subtle, continuous release of its calming scent. These practices can be particularly beneficial for individuals dealing with chronic stress or anxiety disorders.

Beyond its stress-relieving properties, lavender is widely used as a natural sleep aid. Insomnia and poor sleep quality are common issues that can have profound effects on overall health and well-being. Lavender helps address these problems by promoting deeper, more restful sleep. The calming effects of lavender on the nervous system extend to its ability to enhance sleep quality. Linalool, one of the primary components of lavender essential oil, interacts with the brain's neurotransmitters, such as gamma-aminobutyric acid (GABA), which is known for its inhibitory effect on the nervous system. This interaction helps induce a state of relaxation conducive to sleep.

Research supports the use of lavender for improving sleep. A study published in the journal "Holistic Nursing Practice" demonstrated that patients in an intensive care unit who inhaled lavender essential oil experienced significantly better sleep quality compared to those who did not. Similarly, another study found that lavender aromatherapy improved sleep quality and duration in college students with self-reported sleep issues. These findings highlight lavender's potential as a safe and effective alternative to pharmaceutical sleep aids.

Incorporating lavender into a bedtime routine can significantly improve sleep hygiene. Here are some practical ways to use lavender for better sleep:

- **Lavender Essential Oil:** Creating a tranquil atmosphere in the bedroom can be accomplished by adding a few drops of lavender essential oil to a diffuser and allowing it to perform its function. As an alternative, before going to bed, use a blend of lavender essential oil and a carrier oil, such as almond or jojoba oil, that has been diluted and applied to pulse points such as the wrists and the temples respectively.
- **Lavender Pillow Spray:** Create a simple pillow spray by combining distilled water, a small amount of vodka or witch hazel (to help disperse the oil), and several drops of lavender essential oil in a spray bottle. Spritz the pillow and bed linens lightly before going to bed.
- **Lavender Bath:** Taking a warm bath with added lavender essential oil or dried lavender flowers can help relax the muscles and mind, preparing the body for sleep. Adding Epsom salts to the bath can enhance the relaxing effects.

In addition to its benefits for stress and sleep, lavender also possesses mild analgesic and anti-inflammatory properties. Topical applications of lavender oil can help alleviate headaches, muscle pain, and joint stiffness. For instance, a lavender oil massage can reduce muscle tension and provide pain relief. Lavender's antimicrobial properties make it useful for treating minor cuts, burns, and insect bites, promoting healing and reducing the risk of infection.

Lavender can also be used in culinary applications, adding a unique flavor to various dishes while imparting its calming effects. Lavender buds can be used to make herbal teas, infusions, and even baked goods. Lavender tea, in particular, is a soothing beverage that can be enjoyed before bed to enhance relaxation and support sleep. To make lavender tea, steep a teaspoon of dried lavender buds in hot water for 5-10 minutes, strain, and enjoy.

Although lavender is safe for most people, it must be used properly. Before applying essential oils topically, dilute them to avoid skin irritation. Lavender should also be avoided by anyone allergic to Lamiaceae species like mint, rosemary, and sage. Before using lavender essential oil, pregnant and breastfeeding women should see a doctor.

4.5 Turmeric: Anti-Inflammatory Powerhouse

Turmeric (Curcuma longa), often referred to as the "golden spice," is a potent herb widely acclaimed for its anti-inflammatory and antioxidant properties. Originating from Southeast Asia, turmeric has been a staple in traditional Ayurvedic and Chinese medicine for thousands of years. The primary active compound in turmeric, curcumin, is responsible for most of its health benefits. Curcumin has been extensively studied for its ability to modulate inflammation and provide relief from a variety of inflammatory conditions.

The immune system of the body creates inflammation as a natural response to any damage or infection that it encounters. Chronic inflammation, on the other hand, has been linked to a wide range of health issues, including as arthritis, cardiovascular illnesses, diabetes, and even cancer. Curcumin, which is found in turmeric, has the potential to block the activity of various enzymes and cytokines that are involved in the inflammatory process. These enzymes and cytokines include cyclooxygenase-2 (COX-2) and tumor necrosis factor-alpha (TNF-α). Turmeric's anti-inflammatory benefits are mostly contributed to curcumin's function.

Turmeric is famous for treating arthritis. Both osteoarthritis and rheumatoid arthritis cause joint inflammation, discomfort, swelling, and restriction. Research shows that curcumin can significantly reduce arthritic symptoms. A research in "Phytotherapy Research" found that osteoarthritis patients who took curcumin supplements had equal pain and physical function benefits to those using ibuprofen without the gastrointestinal side effects.

The cardiovascular advantages of turmeric are also notable. A key cause of heart disease is chronic inflammation. Anti-inflammatory and antioxidant curcumin reduces oxidative stress, cholesterol, and endothelial function, protecting the heart. The endothelium, which lines blood arteries, is dysfunctional and causes atherosclerosis.

Turmeric inhibits arterial plaque by improving endothelial function.

Additionally advantageous to metabolic health is the use of turmeric. The metabolic syndrome is a cluster of disorders that includes obesity, high blood sugar, high blood pressure, and abnormal cholesterol levels. Chronic inflammation is intimately associated to metabolic syndrome. It has been demonstrated that curcumin can enhance insulin sensitivity, lower blood sugar levels, and facilitate weight loss for individuals. Curcumin supplementation was shown to dramatically lower the chance of acquiring type 2 diabetes in patients who were prediabetic, according to a study that was published in the journal "Diabetes Care."

Another topic that is attracting an increasing amount of attention is the neuroprotective power of turmeric. The development of neurodegenerative illnesses like Alzheimer's and Parkinson's is significantly influenced by neuroinflammation, which plays a significant part in the process. Curcumin is a good candidate for the prevention and therapy of these disorders because of its capacity to both lower inflammation and oxidative stress in the brain, as well as its ability to pass the blood-brain barrier. Curcumin has been shown to have the ability to improve cognitive performance and reduce amyloid plaques in Alzheimer's patients, according to research that was published in the journal "Annals of Indian Academy of Neurology."

Turmeric has antioxidant and anti-inflammatory effects. Curcumin neutralizes free radicals, which harm cells and cause aging and chronic diseases. Turmeric's antioxidants protect cells from oxidative stress and promote health and longevity.

Turmeric's versatility extends to its culinary uses. The spice is a key ingredient in many traditional dishes, particularly in Indian and Southeast Asian cuisines. Its warm, earthy flavor and vibrant yellow color make it a popular addition to curries, soups, and rice dishes. Incorporating turmeric into the diet is a simple way to enjoy its health benefits. However, curcumin's bioavailability is relatively low, meaning that it is not easily absorbed by the body. To enhance absorption, turmeric is often combined with black pepper, which contains piperine, a compound that increases curcumin absorption by up to 2000%.

4.6 Aloe Vera: Skin Soother and Healer

Especially when it comes to skin care, **aloe vera**, also known as **Aloe barbadensis miller**, is a succulent plant that is well-known for its curative and calming effects. Historical records demonstrate that ancient civilizations such as the Egyptians, Greeks, and Chinese exploited aloe vera for its medical advantages. Its use stretches back thousands of years, and it has been well documented. The thick, fleshy leaves of the plant contain a substance that is similar to a gel and is abundant in vitamins, minerals, enzymes, and amino acids, all of which contribute to the effective medicinal benefits of the plant.

One of the primary uses of aloe vera is for treating skin conditions and promoting wound healing. Aloe vera gel has been shown to accelerate the healing of burns, cuts, and abrasions. The gel contains compounds such as glucomannan, a polysaccharide that enhances collagen synthesis and cell regeneration, speeding up the healing process. A study published in the "Journal of Medical Plants Research" found that aloe vera significantly improved the healing of second-degree burns compared to conventional treatments.

Aloe vera's anti-inflammatory and anti-microbial properties make it an effective treatment for various skin conditions, including acne, eczema, and psoriasis. The plant's gel can reduce redness, swelling, and irritation, providing relief from the discomfort associated with these conditions. Its antimicrobial action helps prevent infections, which can complicate skin disorders and delay healing.

The moisturizing properties of aloe vera are another significant benefit, particularly for dry or sensitive skin. Aloe vera gel is composed of approximately 99% water, making it an excellent hydrator. It penetrates the skin easily, providing deep moisture without leaving a greasy residue. This makes aloe vera a popular ingredient in moisturizers, lotions, and other skincare products aimed at hydrating the skin and maintaining its natural moisture balance.

For sunburn relief, aloe vera is unmatched. The cooling sensation of the gel provides immediate relief from the burning and discomfort caused by sun exposure. Its anti-inflammatory properties help to reduce redness and swelling, while its moisturizing effect prevents peeling and promotes faster recovery. Applying fresh aloe vera gel directly from the plant to sunburned skin can soothe pain and support the skin's healing process.

Aloe vera's benefits are not limited to topical applications. The gel can also be ingested to support digestive health. Aloe vera juice is commonly used to treat digestive issues such as acid reflux, irritable bowel syndrome (IBS), and constipation. The plant's enzymes help break down sugars and fats, promoting better digestion and nutrient absorption. Its anti-inflammatory properties can soothe the digestive tract, reducing symptoms of irritation and discomfort. Additionally, aloe vera's natural laxative effect helps to regulate bowel movements and relieve constipation.

To prepare aloe vera juice, it is essential to remove the outer leaf and the yellow latex layer, as these contain compounds that can cause digestive upset. The clear gel inside the leaf can be blended with water or other juices for consumption. It is recommended to start with small amounts to assess tolerance and avoid potential side effects.

Aloe vera is also beneficial for oral health. Its antimicrobial properties can help reduce plaque buildup and combat gum diseases like gingivitis. Using aloe vera gel as a mouthwash can soothe inflamed gums and promote oral hygiene. A study published in the "Journal of Indian Society of Periodontology" found that aloe vera mouthwash was as effective as chlorhexidine in reducing plaque and gingival inflammation.

In addition to its well-documented benefits, aloe vera is easy to grow and maintain, making it a convenient addition to any home apothecary. The plant thrives in warm, sunny environments and requires minimal care. It can be grown in pots indoors or outdoors, making it accessible for those with limited space.

To use aloe vera at home, simply cut a mature leaf from the base of the plant, rinse it to remove any dirt, and slice it open to extract the gel. The fresh gel can be applied directly to the skin or stored in the refrigerator for later use. For internal use, ensure that only the clear gel is consumed, and start with small doses to avoid digestive upset.

The majority of people can consume aloe vera without any adverse effects; nonetheless, it is essential to be aware of the possibility of allergic responses. Before applying aloe vera to broad portions of the skin, it is important to perform a patch test, particularly if you have sensitive skin or a documented history of allergic reactions. In addition, women who are pregnant or breastfeeding, as well as anyone who have specific health conditions, should get the advice of a healthcare expert before consuming aloe vera.

4.7 Peppermint: Digestive and Respiratory Relief

Peppermint (Mentha × piperita) is a widely respected herb known for its distinctive aroma and potent therapeutic properties, particularly in the realms of digestive and respiratory health. A hybrid of watermint and spearmint, peppermint has been used for centuries in traditional medicine across various cultures. Its primary active components, menthol and menthone, confer a range of health benefits, making peppermint an invaluable addition to any natural healing regimen.

The use of peppermint as a digestive aid is one of the most well-known applications of this herb. When it comes to reducing symptoms of indigestion, bloating, and gas, peppermint oil, which is produced from the leaves of the plant, is extremely useful. The antispasmodic qualities of the plant serve to relax the smooth muscles of the gastrointestinal system, which result in a reduction in the frequency and severity of cramps and spasms. This effect is helpful for people who suffer from illnesses such as irritable bowel syndrome (IBS), which is characterized by muscle spasms that lead to discomfort and pain.

Clinical studies have demonstrated the efficacy of peppermint oil in managing IBS symptoms. For instance, a study published in the "Journal of Gastroenterology" found that patients who took enteric-coated peppermint oil capsules experienced significant reductions in abdominal pain, bloating, and gas compared to those who received a placebo. The enteric coating ensures that the peppermint oil is released directly in the intestines, where it can provide the most benefit.

Peppermint tea is another popular way to harness the herb's digestive benefits. The tea can be made by steeping fresh or dried peppermint leaves in hot water for about 5-10 minutes. Drinking peppermint tea after meals can aid digestion, prevent bloating, and promote a sense of overall gastrointestinal comfort. Additionally, the refreshing taste of peppermint tea can help cleanse the palate and reduce feelings of nausea.

Beyond its digestive benefits, peppermint is also highly effective in providing respiratory relief. The menthol in peppermint acts as a natural decongestant, helping to break down mucus and clear the airways. This makes peppermint particularly useful in treating symptoms of colds, sinusitis, and other respiratory conditions. Inhaling steam infused with peppermint oil can provide immediate relief from nasal congestion and improve breathing.

It is necessary to add a few drops of peppermint oil to a bowl of hot water in order to make a peppermint steam inhalation suitable for use. As you lean over the bowl with a towel wrapped over your head to catch the steam, take a few deep breaths and hold them for five to ten minutes. With the aid of this straightforward home remedy, mucus can be loosened, sinus pressure can be reduced, and irritated airways can be soothed.

Peppermint's analgesic and cooling properties also make it an effective remedy for headaches and migraines. Applying diluted peppermint oil to the temples and forehead can help alleviate headache pain. The menthol in peppermint oil induces a cooling sensation that increases blood flow and reduces muscle contractions, providing relief from tension headaches and migraines. A study published in the "International Journal of Phytotherapy and Phytopharmacology" found that peppermint oil was as effective as acetaminophen in reducing headache symptoms.

In addition to topical and aromatic uses, peppermint benefits respiratory health when consumed. Sore throats, coughing, and respiratory function can be improved with peppermint tea. The tea's antispasmodic effects relax respiratory tract muscles, making breathing easier and lowering coughing.

Peppermint is versatile and can be incorporated into various forms, including teas, capsules, essential oils, and topical applications. When using peppermint oil, it is important to dilute it with a carrier oil, such as coconut or almond oil, to prevent skin irritation. A typical dilution ratio is one drop of peppermint oil to a teaspoon of carrier oil. This mixture can be used for massages, compresses, or added to bathwater for a relaxing and therapeutic experience.

A practical example of peppermint's effectiveness is its use in alleviating motion sickness. Peppermint's anti-nausea properties can help prevent the symptoms of motion sickness, such as dizziness, nausea, and vomiting. Chewing on peppermint leaves or drinking peppermint tea before and during travel can help maintain a calm stomach and prevent discomfort.

While peppermint is generally safe for most people, it is important to use it appropriately. High doses of peppermint oil can cause adverse effects, such as heartburn or allergic reactions. Individuals with gastroesophageal reflux disease (GERD) should use peppermint with caution, as it can relax the lower esophageal sphincter and exacerbate symptoms. Pregnant and breastfeeding women should also consult a healthcare provider before using peppermint oil or supplements.

4.8 Dandelion: Detoxification and Liver Support

Dandelion (Taraxacum officinale) is a highly esteemed herb in the world of natural healing, known for its potent detoxifying properties and its ability to support liver health. Often dismissed as a common weed, dandelion boasts a rich history of medicinal use in traditional medicine systems around the globe. Every part of the dandelion plant, from the roots to the flowers, contains valuable nutrients and compounds that contribute to its therapeutic effects.

Dandelion's primary role in natural healing is its ability to promote detoxification. The herb acts as a diuretic, increasing urine production and helping the body eliminate excess fluids and waste products. This diuretic effect is particularly beneficial for individuals suffering from conditions like edema, high blood pressure, and fluid retention. By flushing out toxins through increased urination, dandelion helps maintain the body's internal balance and supports overall health.

In addition to its diuretic properties, dandelion is renowned for its ability to support liver function. The liver is a crucial organ responsible for detoxifying the blood, metabolizing nutrients, and producing bile, which aids in digestion. Dandelion root, in particular, is rich in compounds such as taraxasterol and taraxerol, which stimulate bile production and promote liver regeneration. This makes dandelion an excellent herb for supporting liver health and preventing liver-related disorders.

Studies have shown that dandelion root can protect the liver from damage caused by toxins and oxidative stress. A study published in the "Journal of Ethnopharmacology" found that dandelion root extract significantly reduced liver damage and improved liver function in rats exposed to toxic substances. These findings suggest that dandelion could be a valuable herb for preventing and treating liver diseases such as hepatitis and cirrhosis.

Dandelion's detoxifying and liver-supporting properties also make it an effective herb for promoting digestive health. The increased bile production stimulated by dandelion aids in the digestion and absorption of fats, reducing symptoms of indigestion, bloating, and constipation. Additionally, dandelion's high fiber content supports healthy bowel movements and helps maintain a healthy gut microbiome.

Several different preparations of the herb can be ingested in order to take advantage of the detoxifying and liver-supporting properties that dandelion possesses. The consumption of dandelion tea is among the most common and easily available ways to make use of the herb. To make dandelion tea, soak one to two tablespoons of dried dandelion root or leaves in boiling water for around ten to fifteen minutes. This tea, when consumed up to three times a day, has the potential to maintain healthy liver function, encourage detoxification, and enhance digestion.

Dandelion is also available as a tincture or pill. The medicinal elements of the herb are concentrated and easily absorbed in tinctures. To decide your dosage, visit a doctor or follow the manufacturer's recommendations.

In addition to its internal benefits, dandelion can be used topically to promote skin health. The sap from dandelion stems has been traditionally used to treat skin conditions such as warts, acne, and eczema. The antimicrobial and anti-inflammatory properties of dandelion sap help to reduce skin infections and promote healing. Applying fresh dandelion sap directly to the affected area can provide relief from skin irritations and support the healing process.

Dandelion's nutritional profile is another reason it is highly valued in natural healing. The plant is rich in vitamins A, C, and K, as well as minerals like potassium, calcium, and magnesium. These nutrients contribute to dandelion's overall health benefits, supporting immune function, bone health, and cardiovascular health. Including dandelion greens in salads, soups, and smoothies is a simple way to incorporate these nutrients into your diet.

A practical example of dandelion's effectiveness can be seen in its use as a natural remedy for detoxifying the body after a period of heavy medication or alcohol consumption. For instance, after completing a course of antibiotics, which can strain the liver and disrupt the gut microbiome, a person might use dandelion tea or tincture to help restore liver function and promote the elimination of residual toxins from the body.

It is essential to make sure that dandelion is used appropriately and that you are aware of any potential interactions with drugs, despite the fact that it is generally safe for the majority of individuals. Individuals who are currently taking diuretics, lithium, or specific antibiotics should seek the advice of a healthcare expert prior to consuming dandelion because of the potential for dandelion to interfere with these medical treatments. Furthermore, individuals who suffer from allergies to plants belonging to the Asteraceae family, which includes ragweed, chrysanthemums, marigolds, and daisies, should exercise caution when utilizing dandelion herb.

CHAPTER 5
Herbal Solutions for Specific Health Concerns

5.1 Digestive Health: Herbal Remedies for Common Issues

Digestive health is a cornerstone of overall well-being, as the digestive system is responsible for breaking down food, absorbing nutrients, and eliminating waste. When digestive issues arise, they can significantly impact quality of life. Herbal remedies offer a natural and effective way to address common digestive problems such as indigestion, bloating, gas, constipation, and irritable bowel syndrome (IBS). These remedies have been used for centuries and are supported by both traditional knowledge and modern scientific research.

One of the most widely used herbs for digestive health is **peppermint (Mentha × piperita)**. Peppermint contains menthol, a compound that has antispasmodic properties, helping to relax the smooth muscles of the gastrointestinal tract. This can alleviate symptoms such as bloating, gas, and cramping. Peppermint oil, particularly in enteric-coated capsules, is effective in managing IBS. Enteric-coated capsules ensure that the oil is released in the intestines rather than the stomach, reducing the risk of heartburn. Studies have shown that peppermint oil can significantly reduce the severity of IBS symptoms, making it a valuable remedy for this condition.

Ginger (Zingiber officinale) is another herb that has been used for digestive difficulties for a very long time. Ginger is well-known for its capacity to activate digestive enzymes and bile production, which in turn helps with the digestion of lipids and the general absorption of nutrients. Additionally, it possesses powerful anti-nausea characteristics, which endow it with the ability to effectively alleviate nausea and vomiting that are associated with motion sickness, pregnancy, and chemotherapy. Ginger can be ingested in a number of different forms, including but not limited to fresh, dried, powdered, and infusion forms. Indigestion and nausea can be effectively treated with ginger tea, which is created by steeping fresh ginger slices in hot water. Ginger tea is a simple and efficient cure.

Chamomile (Matricaria chamomilla) has the ability to reduce inflammation and relax the digestive tract. Indigestion, bloating, and gas are all examples of mild digestive problems that can be treated with chamomile tea, which is a typical medication. Chamomile's anti-inflammatory and antispasmodic characteristics assist to calm the muscles of the digestive system, making it an especially beneficial remedy for easing colic in newborns and digestive discomfort in adults. Chamomile is a herb that has been used for centuries. The consumption of chamomile tea following meals has the potential to facilitate digestion and prevent digestive problems.

Fennel (Foeniculum vulgare) is another

herb that has been used traditionally to maintain the health of the digestive system. The seeds of the fennel plant contain a chemical called anethole, which has been shown to relieve bloating and gas in addition to relaxing the muscles of the gastrointestinal tract. The consumption of fennel tea or the chewing of fennel seeds after meals can be beneficial in reducing the symptoms of indigestion and enhancing the general comfort of the digestive system. In addition, fennel is a great treatment for infant colic since it helps to alleviate gas and calms the digestive system.

For those suffering from **constipation, senna (Senna alexandrina)** is a powerful herbal remedy. Senna leaves and pods contain compounds called sennosides, which stimulate bowel movements by irritating the lining of the intestines. While effective, senna should be used sparingly and not for prolonged periods, as it can lead to dependency and disrupt normal bowel function. It is best used as a short-term solution for acute constipation.

Licorice root (Glycyrrhiza glabra) is an effective treatment for digestive conditions that are caused by inflammation. These conditions include gastritis and peptic ulcers. Due to its anti-inflammatory and mucoprotective characteristics, licorice root is able to provide relief to the lining of the intestines and stomach, as well as protect it from further damage. On the other hand, deglycyrrhizinated licorice, also known as DGL, is a type of licorice that has had the glycyrrhizin removed in order to lessen the likelihood of adverse consequences such as elevated blood pressure. In order to improve digestive health and ease symptoms of indigestion and heartburn, it is possible to take chewable tablets or DGL supplements prior to meals.

A practical example of herbal remedies for digestive health is the use of a **digestive tea blend**. Combining herbs like peppermint, ginger, chamomile, and fennel can create a powerful tea that supports overall digestive function. Here is a simple recipe for a **digestive tea blend**:

- 1 teaspoon dried peppermint leaves
- 1 teaspoon dried chamomile flowers
- 1 teaspoon dried ginger root
- 1 teaspoon fennel seeds

Combine the herbs and steep in hot water for 10-15 minutes. Strain and drink after meals to aid digestion and prevent digestive discomfort.

In conclusion, herbal remedies offer a natural and effective approach to managing common digestive issues. By incorporating herbs like peppermint, ginger, chamomile, fennel, senna, and licorice root into daily routines, individuals can support their digestive health and alleviate symptoms such as indigestion, bloating, gas, constipation, and IBS. These time-tested remedies provide a holistic way to maintain digestive wellness and enhance overall quality of life.

5.2 Immune Support: Boosting Your Body's Defenses

When it comes to safeguarding the body from infections and diseases, having a strong immune system is really necessary. Since ancient times, people have relied on herbal medicines to help strengthen and improve immune function. These cures provide a natural method to sustaining health and warding off illness altogether. These herbs include bioactive chemicals that have the ability to boost the immune system, enhance the generation of white blood cells, and provide effects that are antiviral, antibacterial, and anti-inflammatory. In this article, we will discuss some of the most powerful herbs that possess the ability to strengthen the body's defenses and to promote general immunological health.

Echinacea (Echinacea purpurea) is one of the most well-known and extensively investigated herbs. It is through the stimulation of the immune system that echinacea is able to increase the activity of white blood cells, so strengthening the body's capacity to effectively combat illnesses. Furthermore, it is particularly useful in avoiding colds and the flu and in shortening the length of their symptoms. Echinacea, when taken at the first sign of a cold, has been demonstrated to lower the severity of symptoms as well as the length of time they last, according to studies. Tea, tincture, and capsules are all forms of consumption that can be utilized for echinacea.

Elderberry (Sambucus nigra) is another potent immune-boosting herb. The berries and flowers of the elderberry plant are rich in antioxidants and vitamins, particularly vitamin C, which supports immune function. Elderberry has been shown to inhibit the replication of viruses and reduce the severity and duration of cold and flu symptoms. Elderberry syrup, made by simmering the berries with water and honey, is a popular and effective remedy. Studies have demonstrated that elderberry extract can significantly shorten the duration of influenza and reduce the severity of symptoms.

Astragalus (Astragalus membranaceus) is a traditional Chinese herb that is acknowledged for its ability to strengthen the immune system. The immune system is strengthened by the presence of polysaccharides, saponins, and flavonoids in astragalus. These components stimulate the creation of white blood cells and enhance the function of these cells. In addition to this, it possesses adaptogenic qualities, which assist the body in overcoming stress and developing resilience. Astragalus can be consumed in the form of a tea, tincture, or capsules, and it is especially advantageous to utilize it as a preventative measure throughout the spring and fall flu and cold seasons.

Garlic (Allium sativum) is a powerful herb with strong antimicrobial and immune-boosting properties. Allicin, a compound found in garlic, has been shown to enhance the immune response and provide antibacterial, antiviral, and antifungal effects. Regular consumption of garlic can help prevent infections and support overall immune health. Fresh garlic can be added to food, or it can be taken in supplement form. A study published in the "Journal of Nutrition" found that garlic supplementation reduced the incidence and severity of the common cold.

Ginger (Zingiber officinale), in addition to its digestive benefits, is also effective in supporting the immune system. Ginger has anti-inflammatory and antioxidant properties that help to modulate the immune response and protect against oxidative stress. It can also help to clear respiratory infections and reduce symptoms of colds and flu. Ginger tea, made by steeping fresh ginger slices in hot water, is a soothing and effective remedy for boosting immune function and relieving respiratory symptoms.

Turmeric (Curcuma longa) is another herb that is well-known for its immune-enhancing effects. This is mostly owing to the active ingredient curcumin that it contains. Because of its powerful anti-inflammatory and antioxidant properties, curcumin has the potential to improve immune function and provide protection against potential infections. Turmeric, when consumed on a regular basis, has the potential to modify the immune response and lessen the risk of developing chronic diseases. Golden milk is a traditional Ayurvedic beverage that is created with turmeric, milk, and spices. Turmeric can be ingested in the form of golden milk, also known as golden milk, or it can be added to meals.

Licorice root (Glycyrrhiza glabra) is a multipurpose herb. The root of licorice has the ability to increase the production of interferons, which are proteins that are considered to be extremely important in the immunological response to viral infections. In addition to this, it has anti-inflammatory properties, which contribute to the modulation of the immune system and the reduction of the severity of infections. It is possible to consume licorice root in the form of a tea, tincture, or capsules; however, persons who have high blood pressure should exercise caution when consuming it because it has the potential to cause sodium retention and potassium loss.

A practical example of incorporating these herbs into a daily routine for immune support is the preparation of an **immune-boosting herbal tea blend**. This blend can include echinacea, elderberry, astragalus, ginger, and turmeric for a comprehensive immune-boosting effect:

- 1 teaspoon dried echinacea root
- 1 teaspoon dried elderberries
- 1 teaspoon dried astragalus root
- 1 teaspoon fresh ginger slices
- 1 teaspoon turmeric powder

Combine the herbs and simmer in a quart of water for 20-30 minutes. Strain and drink 1-2 cups daily, especially during cold and flu season, to support immune function and prevent infections.

5.3 Mental Wellness: Managing Stress, Anxiety, and Sleep Disorders

Mental wellness is a crucial aspect of overall health, impacting every facet of our lives. Stress, anxiety, and sleep disorders are common issues that can severely affect mental and physical well-being. Herbal remedies offer natural, effective solutions for managing these conditions, providing relief without the side effects often associated with pharmaceutical treatments. Various herbs have been traditionally used to support mental wellness by promoting relaxation, reducing anxiety, and improving sleep quality.

Ashwagandha (Withania somnifera) is a potent adaptogen, reduces stress and anxiety. Naturally occurring adaptogens help the body adapt to stress and preserve balance. Ashwagandha modulates the stress-regulating hypothalamic-pituitary-adrenal (HPA) axis. Ashwagandha has been found to reduce cortisol, the main stress hormone, lowering stress symptoms. It can be used daily in capsules, powders, or tinctures to control stress.

Valerian (Valeriana officinalis) is another herb renowned for its calming effects and ability to promote restful sleep. Valerian root contains compounds such as valerenic acid and valepotriates, which interact with gamma-aminobutyric acid (GABA) receptors in the brain. GABA is a neurotransmitter that induces relaxation and reduces anxiety. Valerian is particularly effective in treating insomnia and improving sleep quality. Drinking valerian tea or taking valerian supplements before bedtime can help individuals fall asleep faster and experience deeper, more restorative sleep.

Lavender (Lavandula angustifolia) is frequently utilized for the purpose of reducing tension and enhancing sleep habits. For the purpose of inducing a state of relaxation, the essential oil of lavender can be inhaled or applied topically. The use of lavender oil has been shown to dramatically lower the levels of anxiety experienced by people who suffer from generalized anxiety disorder, according to research and studies. Additionally, it has been demonstrated that lavender aromatherapy can improve the quality of sleep in a variety of demographics, including patients who are patients in hospitals and people who suffer from insomnia. In the evening, using a diffuser that contains lavender essential oil or adding a few drops of the oil to a bath can be a calming ritual that can be used before going to bed.

Passionflower (Passiflora incarnata) has been used to treat anxiety and sleeplessness. Passionflower's flavonoids and alkaloids reduce anxiety and promote sleep. Passionflower raises brain GABA like valerian. It comes in tea, tincture, and pill form. The "Journal of Clinical Pharmacy and Therapeutics" revealed that passionflower extract reduced anxiety symptoms as well as oxazepam with fewer side effects.

Chamomile (Matricaria chamomilla) is another known soothing herb. Apigenin, a flavonoid in chamomile, binds to brain GABA receptors to relax and reduce anxiety. Many people use chamomile tea to relieve stress and insomnia. Before bed, chamomile tea relaxes the mind and body, making sleep easier. Chamomile extract reduced generalized anxiety disorder symptoms in a "Journal of Clinical Psychopharmacology" study, suggesting it may be a natural anxiolytic.

Lemon balm (Melissa officinalis) has been used for millennia to alleviate anxiety and tension. Lemon balm's rosmarinic acid boosts brain GABA, calming and uplifting. Lemon balm is available in tea, tincture, and capsule form. Combining it with valerian and chamomile is really useful. A research in the "Journal of Herbal Pharmacotherapy" found that lemon balm and valerian improved sleep and anxiety.

Kava (Piper methysticum) is a South Pacific herb known for its powerful anxiolytic effects. The kavalactones in kava interact with GABA receptors in the brain, producing a calming effect without impairing cognitive function. Kava is particularly effective in treating anxiety disorders and has been shown to reduce symptoms of generalized anxiety disorder, social anxiety, and stress-related insomnia. It can be consumed as a tea, tincture, or in capsule form. However, it is important to use kava with caution, as excessive consumption can lead to liver toxicity.

A practical example of incorporating these herbs into a daily routine for mental wellness is the preparation of a **calming herbal tea blend**. This blend can include ashwagandha, valerian, lavender, passionflower, and chamomile for a comprehensive calming effect:

- 1 teaspoon dried ashwagandha root
- 1 teaspoon dried valerian root
- 1 teaspoon dried lavender flowers
- 1 teaspoon dried passionflower
- 1 teaspoon dried chamomile flowers

Combine the herbs and steep in hot water for 10-15 minutes. Strain and drink this tea in the evening to promote relaxation and improve sleep quality.

5.4 Skin and Hair Care: Natural Remedies for Common Conditions

Skin and hair are not only essential for physical appearance but also play crucial roles in protecting the body from environmental hazards. Maintaining their health is vital, and herbal remedies offer natural, effective solutions for various skin and hair conditions. These remedies, rooted in centuries of traditional use, harness the power of nature to promote healing, soothe irritations, and enhance overall vitality.

Aloe Vera (Aloe barbadensis miller) is one of the most versatile and widely used herbs for skin care. Its gel is rich in vitamins, minerals, and amino acids, making it an excellent natural moisturizer and healer. Aloe vera is particularly effective in treating burns, cuts, and other minor wounds due to its anti-inflammatory and antimicrobial properties. It accelerates healing by stimulating collagen production and reducing inflammation. Applying fresh aloe vera gel directly from the plant to the affected area can soothe sunburns, reduce redness, and promote skin regeneration.

Calendula (Calendula officinalis), also known as marigold, is renowned for its skin-soothing and healing properties. The flavonoids and triterpenoids in calendula have anti-inflammatory and antimicrobial effects, making it useful for treating a variety of skin conditions such as eczema, dermatitis, and minor wounds. Calendula-infused oils, creams, and ointments can be applied topically to reduce inflammation, heal skin irritations, and promote overall skin health. A calendula salve can be easily made by infusing dried calendula flowers in olive oil and mixing it with beeswax.

Chamomile (Matricaria chamomilla) is another herb that is gentle yet highly effective for skin care. Chamomile contains azulene, a compound with strong anti-inflammatory and antioxidant properties, which helps to soothe irritated skin and reduce redness. Chamomile is particularly beneficial for sensitive skin and conditions like rosacea and dermatitis. Chamomile tea can be used as a facial rinse to calm inflammation, or chamomile essential oil can be added to skin care products to enhance their soothing effects.

Lavender (Lavandula angustifolia) is celebrated not only for its calming aroma but also for its skin-healing properties. Lavender oil has antiseptic and anti-inflammatory effects, which make it useful for treating acne, reducing scarring, and healing minor cuts and burns. Its antimicrobial properties help prevent infections, while its soothing

qualities reduce irritation and promote relaxation. A few drops of lavender essential oil can be added to carrier oils, creams, or bathwater to benefit the skin.

Tea Tree Oil (Melaleuca alternifolia) is a potent antiseptic and antibacterial agent that is very useful in the treatment of acne and other skin problems caused by bacteria. Tea tree oil contains terpenes that are able to permeate the skin and unblock sebaceous glands, disinfect pores, and dry up blackheads and whiteheads. It is possible to relieve inflammation and prevent future outbreaks by using tea tree oil that has been diluted to regions that are prone to acne. The treatment of fungal infections, such as nail fungus and athlete's foot, is another application for this substance.

Rosehip Seed Oil (Rosa canina) is rich in essential fatty acids and antioxidants, making it an excellent oil for skin rejuvenation and repair. It is particularly effective in reducing the appearance of scars, wrinkles, and hyperpigmentation. The vitamin A and C content in rosehip seed oil promotes collagen production and skin regeneration. Regular application of rosehip seed oil can improve skin texture, elasticity, and tone.

Neem (Azadirachta indica) is a powerful herb that is utilized extensively in Ayurvedic medicine due to its qualities of being anti-inflammatory, anti-fungal, and antibacterial. Both neem oil and neem leaf extracts have been shown to be effective in the treatment of a variety of skin disorders, including acne, eczema, and psoriasis. Neem is beneficial for the skin since it helps to cleanse it, reduce inflammation, and fight off infections. An application of neem oil can be made directly to the skin, and neem leaf powder can be utilized in the formulation of washes and masks.

For hair care, several herbs offer natural solutions to common problems such as dandruff, hair loss, and scalp irritation:

Rosemary (Rosmarinus officinalis) stimulates hair growth and scalp health. Rosemary oil boosts scalp blood flow, promoting hair growth and reducing loss. Its antibacterial qualities prevent dandruff and scalp inflammation. Adding a few drops of rosemary essential oil to shampoo or massaging it into the scalp can improve hair health.

Horsetail (Equisetum arvense) is rich in silica, which strengthens hair strands and promotes hair growth. The minerals in horsetail also help improve the elasticity and texture of hair. Horsetail can be used as a tea rinse or added to hair care products to strengthen and condition the hair.

Amla (Phyllanthus emblica), also known as Indian gooseberry, is a traditional Ayurvedic remedy for hair health. Amla is rich in vitamin C and antioxidants, which nourish the hair follicles, prevent premature graying, and promote hair growth. Amla oil can be massaged into the scalp or amla powder can be used in hair masks to improve hair strength and shine.

Fenugreek (Trigonella foenum-graecum) seeds are another excellent remedy for hair health. Fenugreek seeds are high in protein and nicotinic acid, which help prevent hair loss and stimulate hair growth. Soaking fenugreek seeds overnight and applying the paste to the scalp can reduce dandruff, strengthen hair roots, and promote healthier hair.

A practical example of using these herbs for skin and hair care is the preparation of a **nourishing herbal oil blend**:

* 1 tablespoon dried calendula flowers
* 1 tablespoon dried chamomile flowers
* 1 tablespoon dried lavender flowers
* 1 tablespoon dried rosemary leaves
* 1 cup carrier oil (such as olive oil or jojoba oil)

In a jar made of glass, mixed together the dry herbs and the carrier oil. The jar should be sealed and placed in a warm, sunny location for two to four weeks, with the lid being shaken occasionally. Once the oil has been strained, place it in a bottle made of dark glass. This herbal oil mixture can be applied to the scalp in the form of a massage, used as a treatment for the hair, or used as a soothing oil for skin that is dry and irritable.

5.5 Women's Health: Hormonal Balance and Menstrual Health

Women's health encompasses a wide range of issues, including hormonal balance and menstrual health, which are crucial for overall well-being. Herbal remedies offer natural and effective solutions for managing hormonal fluctuations, alleviating menstrual discomfort, and supporting reproductive health. These remedies have been used for centuries in various traditional medicine systems and are backed by modern scientific research.

Chasteberry (Vitex agnus-castus) is one of the most well-known herbs for supporting hormonal balance in women. It works by regulating the pituitary gland, which helps balance the production of hormones such as progesterone and estrogen. Chasteberry is particularly effective in treating premenstrual syndrome (PMS) symptoms, such as mood swings, breast tenderness, and irritability. Studies have shown that chasteberry can reduce the severity of PMS symptoms and improve overall menstrual health. It is available in various forms, including tinctures, capsules, and teas.

Black Cohosh (Actaea racemosa) is commonly used to alleviate menopausal symptoms and improve hormonal balance. Hot flashes, night sweats, and mood swings are some of the symptoms that can be alleviated by using black cohosh since it includes phytoestrogens, which are substances that mimic the effects of estrogen in the body. The frequency and severity of hot flashes experienced by menopausal women were shown to be greatly reduced by black cohosh, according to a study that was published in the journal "Menopause." When it comes to supporting hormonal health throughout menopause, black cohosh can be consumed in the form of a tincture, pill, or loose tea.

Red Clover (Trifolium pratense) is rich in isoflavones, which are plant-based compounds that mimic estrogen in the body. This makes red clover an effective remedy for managing menopausal symptoms and supporting overall hormonal balance. Red clover can help reduce hot flashes, improve bone density, and promote cardiovascular health. It can be consumed as a tea or taken in supplement form. Red clover's gentle, estrogen-like effects make it a popular choice for women seeking natural alternatives to hormone replacement therapy.

Dong Quai (Angelica sinensis), often referred to as "female ginseng," is a traditional Chinese herb known for its ability to support menstrual and reproductive health. Dong quai helps regulate the menstrual cycle, reduce menstrual cramps, and alleviate symptoms of PMS. It also improves blood flow and supports overall vitality. Dong quai can be taken as a tincture, capsule, or tea. Its balancing effects on the female reproductive system make it a valuable herb for women experiencing irregular menstrual cycles or other menstrual disorders.

Ginger (Zingiber officinale) is not only beneficial for digestive health but also for alleviating menstrual pain. Ginger has anti-inflammatory and analgesic properties that can reduce menstrual cramps and discomfort. A study published in "Pain Medicine" found that ginger was as effective as ibuprofen in relieving menstrual pain. Drinking ginger tea or taking ginger supplements during menstruation can help alleviate cramps and promote a more comfortable menstrual experience.

Raspberry Leaf (Rubus idaeus) is a traditional herb used to support uterine health and ease menstrual symptoms. Raspberry leaf is rich in vitamins and minerals, including iron, calcium, and magnesium, which help strengthen the uterine muscles and reduce menstrual cramps. It also helps regulate the menstrual cycle and support overall reproductive health. Raspberry leaf tea is a popular and effective way to consume this herb. Drinking raspberry leaf tea regularly can promote a healthy menstrual cycle and alleviate PMS symptoms.

One other effective treatment for women's health is evening primrose oil, which comes from the **Oenothera biennis** plant. It has a high concentration of gamma-linolenic acid (GLA), which is an important fatty acid that serves to reduce inflammation and maintain hormonal equilibrium. When it comes to treating symptoms of premenstrual syndrome (PMS), such as breast discomfort, mood swings, and bloating, evening primrose oil is very effective. Additionally, it has the potential to enhance the health of the skin and alleviate the symptoms of eczema and acne. Evening primrose oil is available in capsule form and can be consumed on a regular basis to improve hormonal balance and menstrual health.

Adaptogenic **Maca Root (Lepidium meyenii)** balances hormones and boosts energy. Maca root affects hormone generation and secretion in the endocrine system. For women with hormonal imbalances from menopause, PMS, or PCOS, it is very helpful. You can take maca root powder, pill, or tincture. Its adaptogenic characteristics aid stress management and hormonal balance.

A practical example of using these herbs

for hormonal balance and menstrual health is the preparation of a **herbal tea blend**:

- 1 teaspoon dried chasteberry
- 1 teaspoon dried red clover
- 1 teaspoon dried raspberry leaf
- 1 teaspoon dried dong quai
- 1 teaspoon dried ginger root

Combine the herbs and steep in hot water for 10-15 minutes. Strain and drink this tea daily to support hormonal balance and alleviate menstrual discomfort.

In addition to these herbs, lifestyle practices such as regular exercise, a balanced diet, adequate hydration, and stress management are crucial for maintaining hormonal health and supporting the menstrual cycle. Incorporating these herbs into daily routines, along with healthy lifestyle practices, can provide comprehensive support for women's hormonal and menstrual health.

5.6 Men's Health: Prostate Support and Vitality Enhancement

Men's health encompasses a variety of issues, with prostate health and vitality being among the most critical. Herbal remedies offer natural, effective solutions for supporting prostate function, enhancing vitality, and promoting overall well-being. These remedies have been utilized for centuries in traditional medicine systems and are increasingly supported by scientific research.

Saw Palmetto (Serenoa repens) is highly regarded as one of the most effective medicines for promoting healthy prostate function. The benign prostatic hyperplasia (BPH) condition, which is characterized by an enlarged prostate and is frequent in elderly men, is treated with this medication with great success. Inhibiting the enzyme 5-alpha-reductase, which is responsible for the conversion of testosterone into dihydrotestosterone (DHT), a hormone that has a role in the development of the prostate, is how saw palmetto can be effective. Studies have demonstrated that saw palmetto can alleviate bladder symptoms that are linked with benign prostatic hyperplasia (BPH), such as the need to urinate frequently and the difficulty in beginning to urinate. Saw palmetto can be consumed in a number of different ways, including teas, tinctures, and capsules from the manufacturer.

Pygeum (Prunus africana) is another herb beneficial for prostate health. Extracts from the bark of the African cherry tree have been used traditionally to treat urinary and prostate issues. Pygeum has anti-inflammatory properties and helps reduce the symptoms of BPH by decreasing prostate inflammation and improving urinary flow. Research has shown that pygeum can effectively reduce nocturia (frequent nighttime urination) and improve overall urinary function. Pygeum supplements are widely available and can be incorporated into a daily health regimen for prostate support.

Nettle Root (Urtica dioica) is commonly used in combination with other herbs like saw palmetto and pygeum to support prostate health. Nettle root helps reduce the symptoms of BPH by inhibiting the binding of DHT to androgen receptors in the prostate. This action helps to reduce prostate growth and alleviate urinary symptoms. Nettle root also has anti-inflammatory and diuretic properties, which further support urinary health. Nettle root can be consumed as a tea, tincture, or in capsule form.

Pumpkin Seed (Cucurbita pepo) extract is rich in essential fatty acids, antioxidants, and phytosterols, which support prostate health and reduce the symptoms of BPH. Pumpkin seed oil has been shown to improve urinary function and reduce inflammation in the prostate. The high zinc content in pumpkin seeds is also beneficial for maintaining healthy testosterone levels and supporting overall reproductive health. Consuming pumpkin seeds as a snack or taking pumpkin seed oil supplements can help support prostate function and reduce urinary symptoms.

Ginseng (Panax ginseng) is a well-known adaptogen that helps enhance vitality and overall well-being. Ginseng has been traditionally used to improve physical and mental performance, boost energy levels, and support immune function. It is particularly beneficial for men experiencing fatigue, stress, and low libido. Ginseng works by regulating the endocrine system and enhancing the body's resistance to stress. Studies have shown that ginseng can improve erectile function and increase sexual satisfaction. Ginseng can be consumed as a tea, tincture, or in supplement form to boost vitality and overall health.

Tribulus (Tribulus terrestris) is a herb commonly used to enhance male vitality and support healthy testosterone levels. Tribulus has been shown to increase libido, improve sexual performance, and support muscle growth and physical strength. It works by stimulating the production of luteinizing hormone, which in turn increases testosterone levels. Tribulus can be taken as a supplement or in tea form to support reproductive health and enhance vitality.

Maca Root (Lepidium meyenii) is another powerful adaptogen known for its ability to enhance energy, stamina, and sexual health. Maca root helps regulate hormone levels, improve libido, and increase fertility. Studies have shown that maca root can improve sexual desire and performance, making it a popular choice for men seeking to enhance their vitality. Maca root can be taken as a powder, capsule, or tincture and can be easily incorporated into daily routines.

A practical example of using these herbs for prostate support and vitality enhancement is the preparation of a **herbal supplement blend:**

* 1 teaspoon saw palmetto extract
* 1 teaspoon pygeum extract
* 1 teaspoon nettle root extract
* 1 teaspoon pumpkin seed oil
* 1 teaspoon ginseng extract
* 1 teaspoon tribulus extract
* 1 teaspoon maca root powder

Combine the extracts and powder in a glass of water or juice and drink daily to support prostate health and enhance vitality.

In addition to these herbs, lifestyle practices such as regular exercise, a balanced diet, adequate hydration, and stress management are crucial for maintaining prostate health and overall vitality. Incorporating these herbs into daily routines, along with healthy lifestyle practices, can provide comprehensive support for men's health.

5.7 Children's Health: Safe Herbal Treatments for All Ages

Children's health is a priority for every parent, and using safe, natural herbal remedies can be an effective way to support their well-being. Herbal treatments offer gentle solutions for common childhood ailments, such as colds, digestive issues, skin irritations, and anxiety, without the harsh side effects often associated with pharmaceuticals. These remedies have been used for generations and can provide comfort and healing for children of all ages.

Chamomile (Matricaria chamomilla) is one of the most gentle and versatile herbs suitable for children. Its calming properties make it ideal for treating anxiety, restlessness, and sleep disturbances. Chamomile tea can help soothe an upset stomach, alleviate colic, and reduce symptoms of indigestion. For teething babies, a cooled chamomile tea bag can be given to chew on, providing relief from gum pain. Chamomile can also be used as a topical wash to treat skin irritations and rashes. Its anti-inflammatory and antimicrobial properties help soothe and heal the skin.

Ginger (Zingiber officinale) is another plant that is both safe and beneficial for children, particularly for children who have stomach disorders. Indigestion, nausea, and motion sickness are among symptoms that can be alleviated by ginger. In order to assist in the settlement of children's tummies, a mild ginger tea that is prepared by steeping a tiny amount of fresh ginger in hot water can be administered to the children. In addition, ginger possesses anti-inflammatory qualities, which makes it an effective remedy for the treatment of colds and sore throats. It is possible to alleviate a sore throat and reduce coughing by using honey that has been infused with ginger.

Elderberry (Sambucus nigra) is well-known for its immune-enhancing characteristics and is especially beneficial in preventing and treating several illnesses, including the common cold and influenza. The administration of elderberry syrup to children can serve as a preventative measure during the cold and flu season, or it can be administered at the initial symptom of disease. Elderberry contains a high concentration of antioxidants and vitamins, both of which provide support to the immune system and aid in the fight against illnesses. Elderberry has been demonstrated in studies to lessen the severity and duration of symptoms associated with the common cold and influenza. Gummies made from elderberries or elderberry syrup are two common forms that children love consuming.

Peppermint (Mentha × piperita) is a helpful herb for relieving digestive discomfort and respiratory issues in children. Pepper-

mint tea can alleviate symptoms of gas, bloating, and indigestion. The menthol in peppermint also acts as a natural decongestant, making it useful for treating colds and sinus congestion. Inhaling steam from a bowl of hot water with a few drops of peppermint essential oil can help clear nasal passages and reduce coughing. Peppermint should be used cautiously in young children, and it is best to consult with a healthcare provider before use.

Calendula (Calendula officinalis) is an excellent herb for treating skin conditions in children. Its anti-inflammatory and antimicrobial properties make it effective for healing cuts, scrapes, and rashes. Calendula-infused oil or cream can be applied to the skin to soothe diaper rash, eczema, and other irritations. Calendula can also be used as a gentle eye wash to treat conjunctivitis (pink eye) and other eye irritations.

Fennel (Foeniculum vulgare) is a gentle herb for infant and child colic and digestive disorders. Fennel tea relaxes gastrointestinal muscles, reducing gas and bloating. Fennel tea can assist nursing moms' babies through breast milk. Fennel's expectorant qualities assist clear mucus from the airways, treating coughs and respiratory congestion.

Lavender (Lavandula angustifolia) is known for its calming and soothing effects, making it an ideal herb for treating anxiety and sleep disturbances in children. Lavender essential oil can be diffused in the child's room or added to a warm bath to promote relaxation and better sleep. Lavender can also be used in a massage oil to calm an anxious or restless child. Its gentle aroma helps create a peaceful environment conducive to rest and relaxation.

Licorice Root (Glycyrrhiza glabra) is beneficial for treating sore throats and coughs in children. It has soothing, anti-inflammatory, and antimicrobial properties that help reduce throat irritation and fight infections. Licorice root tea or a glycerite (a sweet, alcohol-free extract) can be given to children to soothe a sore throat and reduce coughing. However, licorice should be used with caution and not for extended periods, as it can affect blood pressure and potassium levels.

A practical example of incorporating these herbs into a child's routine is the preparation of a **soothing herbal tea blend**:

* 1 teaspoon dried chamomile flowers
* 1 teaspoon dried fennel seeds
* 1 teaspoon dried peppermint leaves (for children over five years old)

Combine the herbs and steep in hot water for 5-10 minutes. Strain and allow the tea to cool to a safe temperature. This gentle tea can be given to children to relieve digestive discomfort, reduce anxiety, and promote relaxation.

In addition to herbal remedies, maintaining a healthy lifestyle is crucial for children's overall well-being. Ensuring a balanced diet, regular physical activity, adequate hydration, and sufficient sleep can help support their immune system and overall health.

5.8 Chronic Conditions: Managing Long-Term Health Issues

Managing chronic conditions often requires a comprehensive approach that includes lifestyle changes, medication, and complementary therapies. Herbal remedies can play a significant role in supporting long-term health and alleviating symptoms associated with chronic illnesses. These remedies, which have been utilized for centuries, offer natural, gentle, and effective options for managing a variety of chronic conditions, from cardiovascular diseases to diabetes and arthritis.

Turmeric (Curcuma longa) is a potent anti-inflammatory herb that is commonly used to reduce chronic inflammation, which is a prevalent underlying factor in many chronic illnesses. There is evidence that curcumin, the active component of turmeric, can alleviate symptoms of disorders such as arthritis, inflammatory bowel disease, and cardiovascular diseases. Curcumin has been found to lower inflammation and oxidative stress. According to the findings of a study that was published in the "Journal of Alternative and Complementary Medicine," patients who suffered from osteoarthritis had a considerable reduction in pain and an improvement in their function when they took curcumin supplements. Consuming turmeric in the form of a spice in food, taking it as a supplement, or brewing it into a tea are all viable options.

Ginger (Zingiber officinale), another potent anti-inflammatory herb, is particularly effective for managing chronic pain and gastrointestinal issues. Ginger has been shown to reduce pain and improve mobility in people with osteoarthritis and rheumatoid arthritis. Its digestive benefits also make it useful for managing chronic conditions such as irritable bowel syndrome (IBS) and dyspepsia. Drinking ginger tea or taking ginger supplements can provide significant relief from chronic pain and digestive discomfort.

Garlic (Allium sativum) is known for its cardiovascular benefits, making it an excellent herb for managing chronic conditions related to heart health. Garlic has been shown to lower blood pressure, reduce cholesterol levels, and improve overall heart function. These effects are primarily due to the presence of allicin, a sulfur-containing compound with potent antioxidant and anti-inflammatory properties. Regular consumption of garlic, whether raw, cooked, or in supplement form, can help manage hypertension and reduce the risk of heart disease.

Cinnamon (Cinnamomum verum): there are many health benefits associated with cinnamon, including the management of metabolic syndrome and diabetes. An increase in insulin sensitivity, a decrease in blood sugar levels, and a reduction in the risk factors associated with diabetes have all been demonstrated outcomes of cinnamon use. Cinnamon supplementation was found to improve blood glucose control in patients with type 2 diabetes, according to a study that was published in the journal Disease Care. Through the addition of cinnamon to foods and beverages, as well as through the consumption of cinnamon in supplement form, cinnamon can be easily introduced into a diet.

Milk Thistle (Silybum marianum) is a valuable herb for liver health, which is essential for managing chronic conditions such as hepatitis and cirrhosis. The active compound in milk thistle, silymarin, has hepatoprotective properties that help regenerate liver cells, reduce inflammation, and protect the liver from toxins. Milk thistle can be taken as a supplement or brewed into a tea to support liver function and overall detoxification.

Hawthorn (Crataegus spp.) is a herb that is used to promote heart health and to manage chronic cardiovascular problems. Several studies have demonstrated that hawthorn can enhance blood flow, lower blood pressure, and strengthen the muscle of the heart. Protecting the heart from oxidative stress and inflammation is made possible by the antioxidant qualities of this substance. For the purpose of promoting cardiovascular health and managing illnesses such as hypertension and congestive heart failure, hawthorn can be consumed in the form of a tea, tincture, or capsules.

Aloe Vera (Aloe barbadensis miller) is effective for managing chronic skin conditions such as psoriasis, eczema, and dermatitis. Aloe vera gel, applied topically, can soothe inflammation, reduce itching, and promote healing. Its antimicrobial properties also help prevent infections. Drinking aloe vera juice can support overall digestive health and help manage conditions like irritable bowel syndrome (IBS) and acid reflux.

Ashwagandha (Withania somnifera) reduces chronic stress and exhaustion typical of many chronic illnesses. Ashwagandha lowers cortisol, boosts resilience, and boosts vitality. It helps manage chronic fatigue syndrome and fibromyalgia. Ashwagandha can be used as a supplement, tincture, powder, or in smoothies or drinks.

A practical example of using these herbs for managing chronic conditions is the preparation of a daily herbal supplement regimen:

- **Turmeric:** 500-1000 mg of curcumin extract with black pepper (to enhance absorption) taken daily to reduce inflammation.
- **Ginger:** 500 mg of ginger extract taken twice daily to alleviate pain and support digestion.
- **Garlic:** One clove of raw garlic or 600-1200 mg of aged garlic extract taken daily to support heart health.
- **Cinnamon:** 1-2 grams of cinnamon powder or 500 mg of cinnamon extract taken daily to manage blood sugar levels.
- **Milk Thistle:** 200-400 mg of silymarin taken daily to support liver health.
- **Hawthorn:** 300-600 mg of hawthorn extract taken daily to support cardiovascular health.
- **Aloe Vera:** 30 ml of aloe vera juice taken daily to support digestive health and applied topically as needed for skin conditions.

- **Ashwagandha:** 300-500 mg of ashwagandha extract taken daily to reduce stress and improve energy levels.

In addition to these herbal remedies, maintaining a healthy lifestyle is crucial for managing chronic conditions. This includes a balanced diet, regular exercise, adequate hydration, and stress management techniques such as mindfulness and meditation.

Herbal remedies offer a natural and effective approach to managing chronic conditions, providing support for long-term health and well-being. By incorporating herbs such as turmeric, ginger, garlic, cinnamon, milk thistle, hawthorn, aloe vera, and ashwagandha into daily routines, individuals can alleviate symptoms, enhance vitality, and improve their overall quality of life. These time-tested remedies provide a holistic way to manage chronic health issues, leveraging the power of nature to support and maintain long-term health.

CHAPTER 6
Herbal Recipes for Everyday Health

Herbal Teas and Infusions

Calming Chamomile Lavender Tea

Preparation Time: 5 minutes   **Cooking Time:** 10 minutes   **Servings:** 2

INGREDIENTS:

- 2 teaspoons dried chamomile flowers
- 1 teaspoon dried lavender flowers
- 2 cups water
- Honey or lemon (optional)

DIRECTIONS:

1. Bring 2 cups of water to a boil in a small pot.
2. Add the dried chamomile and lavender flowers to the boiling water.
3. Reduce the heat and let the mixture simmer for 10 minutes.
4. Remove from heat and strain the tea into cups.
5. Add honey or lemon if desired, and enjoy your calming tea.

Nutritional Values: Calories: 2; Total Fat: 0g; Saturated Fat: 0g; Sodium: 4mg; Total Carbohydrates: 1g; Dietary Fiber: 0g; Protein: 0g; Potassium: 21mg

Digestive Ginger Mint Tea

Preparation Time: 5 minutes   **Cooking Time:** 10 minutes   **Servings:** 2

INGREDIENTS:

- 1 teaspoon fresh ginger, grated
- 1 teaspoon dried peppermint leaves
- 2 cups water
- Honey (optional)

DIRECTIONS:

1. Boil 2 cups of water in a pot.
2. Add the grated ginger and dried peppermint leaves to the boiling water.
3. Reduce the heat and let the mixture simmer for 10 minutes.
4. Strain the tea into cups.
5. Sweeten with honey if desired, and enjoy your soothing digestive tea.

Nutritional Values: Calories: 5; Total Fat: 0g; Saturated Fat: 0g; Sodium: 5mg; Total Carbohydrates: 1g; Dietary Fiber: 0g; Protein: 0g; Potassium: 24mg

Immune-Boosting Elderberry Echinacea Infusion

Preparation Time: 5 minutes   **Cooking Time:** 15 minutes   **Servings:** 2

INGREDIENTS:

- 2 teaspoons dried elderberries
- 1 teaspoon dried echinacea root
- 2 cups water
- Lemon or honey (optional)

DIRECTIONS:

1. Bring 2 cups of water to a boil in a small pot.
2. Add the dried elderberries and echinacea root to the boiling water.
3. Reduce the heat and let the mixture simmer for 15 minutes.
4. Remove from heat and strain the infusion into cups.
5. Add lemon or honey if desired, and enjoy your immune-boosting infusion.

Nutritional Values: Calories: 10; Total Fat: 0g; Saturated Fat: 0g; Sodium: 3mg; Total Carbohydrates: 2g; Dietary Fiber: 0g; Protein: 0g; Potassium: 33mg

Detoxifying Dandelion Nettle Tea

Preparation Time: 5 minutes   **Cooking Time:** 10 minutes   **Servings:** 2

INGREDIENTS:

- 1 teaspoon dried dandelion root
- 1 teaspoon dried nettle leaves
- 2 cups water
- Lemon (optional)

DIRECTIONS:

1. Boil 2 cups of water in a pot.
2. Add the dried dandelion root and nettle leaves to the boiling water.
3. Reduce the heat and let the mixture simmer for 10 minutes.
4. Strain the tea into cups.
5. Add lemon if desired, and enjoy your detoxifying tea.

Nutritional Values: Calories: 7; Total Fat: 0g; Saturated Fat: 0g; Sodium: 6mg; Total Carbohydrates: 2g; Dietary Fiber: 0g; Protein: 0g; Potassium: 40mg

Relaxing Lemon Balm Passionflower Tea

Preparation Time: 5 minutes   **Cooking Time:** 10 minutes   **Servings:** 2

INGREDIENTS:

- 1 teaspoon dried lemon balm leaves
- 1 teaspoon dried passionflower
- 2 cups water
- Honey (optional)

DIRECTIONS:

1. Bring 2 cups of water to a boil in a small pot.
2. Add the dried lemon balm and passionflower to the boiling water.
3. Reduce the heat and let the mixture simmer for 10 minutes.
4. Remove from heat and strain the tea into cups.
5. Sweeten with honey if desired, and enjoy your relaxing tea.

Nutritional Values: Calories: 3; Total Fat: 0g; Saturated Fat: 0g; Sodium: 2mg; Total Carbohydrates: 1g; Dietary Fiber: 0g; Protein: 0g; Potassium: 18mg

Tinctures and Extracts

Herbal tinctures are concentrated liquid extracts made from herbs and alcohol, which capture the potent medicinal properties of the herbs in a highly effective and easily absorbable form. They are an essential component of herbal medicine due to their convenience, potency, and long shelf life. Tinctures can be made from a wide range of herbs to address various health concerns, including boosting the immune system, alleviating digestive issues, reducing inflammation, and promoting relaxation. The process of making tinctures is straightforward, and with a few basic supplies and some patience, you can create your own powerful herbal remedies at home.

To begin, it is crucial to select high-quality herbs, whether fresh or dried. Fresh herbs are ideal for their vibrant potency, but dried herbs can also be used effectively. The alcohol used in tinctures acts as a solvent, extracting the beneficial compounds from the plant material. Typically, 80-proof vodka or brandy is used, as they strike a good balance between potency and taste. The basic method involves combining the herbs and alcohol in a glass jar, sealing it tightly, and storing it in a cool, dark place for several weeks. During this time, the jar is shaken daily to aid in the extraction process. After 4-6 weeks, the mixture is strained, and the liquid tincture is transferred to dark glass bottles for storage.

Using herbal tinctures is both simple and versatile. They can be taken directly under the tongue for rapid absorption or diluted in water, juice, or tea to mask their sometimes strong taste. The dosage of tinctures can vary depending on the herb and the intended use, but a common guideline is to take 1-2 droppers full (approximately 30-60 drops) up to three times daily. It is important to follow specific recommendations for each herb and consult with a healthcare provider, especially when using tinctures for chronic conditions or in combination with other medications.

The benefits of making and using herbal tinctures extend beyond their practical applications. The process of creating tinctures fosters a deeper connection with the plants and a greater understanding of their healing properties. It also allows for customization, enabling you to tailor remedies to your specific health needs. Furthermore, making tinctures at home ensures that you have control over the quality and purity of the ingredients, avoiding the additives and preservatives often found in commercial products.

In summary, herbal tinctures are a powerful, versatile, and accessible form of natural medicine. By learning how to make and use tinctures, you can enhance your health regimen with customized, high-quality herbal extracts. This not only empowers you to take charge of your health but also connects you to the time-honored traditions of herbal medicine. Whether you are new to herbal remedies or an experienced practitioner, the knowledge and skills gained from tincture-making can provide lasting benefits for your well-being.

Echinacea Tincture

Preparation Time: 15 minutes   **Servings:** Makes about 2 cups

INGREDIENTS:

* 1 cup dried echinacea root
* 2 cups 80-proof vodka or brandy

DIRECTIONS:

1. Place the dried echinacea root in a clean, dry glass jar.
2. Pour the vodka or brandy over the echinacea root, ensuring the root is fully submerged.
3. Seal the jar tightly and store it in a cool, dark place.
4. Shake the jar daily for 4-6 weeks to help extract the beneficial compounds.
5. After 4-6 weeks, strain the mixture through a fine mesh strainer or cheesecloth into a clean jar, discarding the plant material.
6. Store the finished tincture in a dark glass bottle, and label it with the date and contents.
7. To use, take 1-2 droppers full (about 30-60 drops) of the tincture in water or juice, up to three times daily.

Valerian Root Tincture

Preparation Time: 15 minutes   **Servings:** Makes about 2 cups

INGREDIENTS:

* 1 cup dried valerian root
* 2 cups 80-proof vodka or brandy

DIRECTIONS:

1. Place the dried valerian root in a clean, dry glass jar.
2. Pour the vodka or brandy over the valerian root, ensuring the root is fully covered.
3. Seal the jar tightly and store it in a cool, dark place.
4. Shake the jar daily for 4-6 weeks to extract the active compounds.
5. After 4-6 weeks, strain the mixture through a fine mesh strainer or cheesecloth into a clean jar, discarding the plant material.
6. Transfer the tincture to dark glass bottles and label them with the date and contents.
7. To use, take 1-2 droppers full (about 30-60 drops) of the tincture in water or juice, 30 minutes before bedtime.

Lemon Balm Tincture

Preparation Time: 15 minutes　　　**Servings:** Makes about 2 cups

INGREDIENTS:

- 1 cup fresh lemon balm leaves (or 1/2 cup dried leaves)
- 2 cups 80-proof vodka or brandy

DIRECTIONS:

1. Place the fresh or dried lemon balm leaves in a clean, dry glass jar.
2. Pour the vodka or brandy over the lemon balm, ensuring the leaves are fully submerged.
3. Seal the jar tightly and store it in a cool, dark place.
4. Shake the jar daily for 4-6 weeks to extract the herbal compounds.
5. After 4-6 weeks, strain the mixture through a fine mesh strainer or cheesecloth into a clean jar, discarding the plant material.
6. Store the finished tincture in dark glass bottles and label them with the date and contents.
7. To use, take 1-2 droppers full (about 30-60 drops) of the tincture in water or juice, up to three times daily.

Ginger Tincture

Preparation Time: 15 minutes　　　**Servings:** Makes about 2 cups

INGREDIENTS:

- 1 cup fresh ginger root, grated (or 1/2 cup dried ginger root)
- 2 cups 80-proof vodka or brandy

DIRECTIONS:

1. Place the grated fresh ginger root or dried ginger root in a clean, dry glass jar.
2. Pour the vodka or brandy over the ginger, ensuring the ginger is fully submerged.
3. Seal the jar tightly and store it in a cool, dark place.
4. Shake the jar daily for 4-6 weeks to extract the active compounds.
5. After 4-6 weeks, strain the mixture through a fine mesh strainer or cheesecloth into a clean jar, discarding the plant material.
6. Transfer the tincture to dark glass bottles and label them with the date and contents.
7. To use, take 1-2 droppers full (about 30-60 drops) of the tincture in water or juice, up to three times daily.

Peppermint Tincture

Preparation Time: 15 minutes   **Servings:** Makes about 2 cups

INGREDIENTS:

- 1 cup fresh peppermint leaves (or 1/2 cup dried leaves)
- 2 cups 80-proof vodka or brandy

DIRECTIONS:

1. Place the fresh or dried peppermint leaves in a clean, dry glass jar.
2. Pour the vodka or brandy over the peppermint, ensuring the leaves are fully submerged.
3. Seal the jar tightly and store it in a cool, dark place.
4. Shake the jar daily for 4-6 weeks to extract the herbal compounds.
5. After 4-6 weeks, strain the mixture through a fine mesh strainer or cheesecloth into a clean jar, discarding the plant material.
6. Store the finished tincture in dark glass bottles and label them with the date and contents.
7. To use, take 1-2 droppers full (about 30-60 drops) of the tincture in water or juice, up to three times daily.

Calendula Healing Salve

Preparation Time: 45 minutes   **Servings:** Makes about 2 cups

INGREDIENTS:

- 1 cup dried calendula flowers
- 1 cup olive oil
- 1/4 cup beeswax
- 10 drops lavender essential oil (optional)

DIRECTIONS:

1. Combine the dried calendula flowers and olive oil in a double boiler.
2. Simmer gently over low heat for 30 minutes, stirring occasionally.
3. Strain the mixture through a cheesecloth or fine mesh strainer into a clean, dry container.
4. Return the infused oil to the double boiler and add the beeswax.
5. Heat gently, stirring until the beeswax is completely melted.
6. Remove from heat and add the lavender essential oil, if using.
7. Pour the mixture into small, sterilized jars or tins and allow it to cool and solidify before sealing.
8. Use the salve to soothe cuts, scrapes, and minor skin irritations.

Arnica Muscle Relief Balm

Preparation Time: 45 minutes   **Servings:** Makes about 2 cups

INGREDIENTS:

- 1 cup dried arnica flowers
- 1 cup coconut oil
- 1/4 cup beeswax
- 10 drops peppermint essential oil (optional)

DIRECTIONS:

1. Place the dried arnica flowers and coconut oil in a double boiler.
2. Simmer gently over low heat for 30 minutes, stirring occasionally.
3. Strain the mixture through a cheesecloth or fine mesh strainer into a clean, dry container.
4. Return the infused oil to the double boiler and add the beeswax.
5. Heat gently, stirring until the beeswax is completely melted.
6. Remove from heat and add the peppermint essential oil, if using.
7. Pour the mixture into small, sterilized jars or tins and allow it to cool and solidify before sealing.
8. Apply the balm to sore muscles and joints for relief from pain and inflammation.

Lavender Chamomile Sleep Balm

Preparation Time: 45 minutes   **Servings:** Makes about 2 cups

INGREDIENTS:

- 1/2 cup dried lavender flowers
- 1/2 cup dried chamomile flowers
- 1 cup almond oil
- 1/4 cup beeswax
- 10 drops lavender essential oil

DIRECTIONS:

1. Combine the dried lavender and chamomile flowers with almond oil in a double boiler.
2. Simmer gently over low heat for 30 minutes, stirring occasionally.
3. Strain the mixture through a cheesecloth or fine mesh strainer into a clean, dry container.
4. Return the infused oil to the double boiler and add the beeswax.
5. Heat gently, stirring until the beeswax is completely melted.
6. Remove from heat and add the lavender essential oil.
7. Pour the mixture into small, sterilized jars or tins and allow it to cool and solidify before sealing.
8. Apply the balm to temples, wrists, or chest before bedtime to promote relaxation and sleep.

Comfrey Healing Balm

Preparation Time: 45 minutes   **Servings:** Makes about 2 cups

INGREDIENTS:

- 1 cup dried comfrey leaves
- 1 cup olive oil
- 1/4 cup beeswax
- 10 drops tea tree essential oil (optional)

DIRECTIONS:

1. Place the dried comfrey leaves and olive oil in a double boiler.
2. Simmer gently over low heat for 30 minutes, stirring occasionally.
3. Strain the mixture through a cheesecloth or fine mesh strainer into a clean, dry container.
4. Return the infused oil to the double boiler and add the beeswax.
5. Heat gently, stirring until the beeswax is completely melted.
6. Remove from heat and add the tea tree essential oil, if using.
7. Pour the mixture into small, sterilized jars or tins and allow it to cool and solidify before sealing.
8. Use the balm to heal bruises, sprains, and minor skin injuries.

Peppermint Cooling Foot Balm

Preparation Time: 45 minutes   **Servings:** Makes about 2 cups

INGREDIENTS:

- 1/2 cup dried peppermint leaves
- 1/2 cup dried calendula flowers
- 1 cup coconut oil
- 1/4 cup beeswax
- 10 drops peppermint essential oil

DIRECTIONS:

1. Combine the dried peppermint leaves and calendula flowers with coconut oil in a double boiler.
2. Simmer gently over low heat for 30 minutes, stirring occasionally.
3. Strain the mixture through a cheesecloth or fine mesh strainer into a clean, dry container.
4. Return the infused oil to the double boiler and add the beeswax.
5. Heat gently, stirring until the beeswax is completely melted.
6. Remove from heat and add the peppermint essential oil.
7. Pour the mixture into small, sterilized jars or tins and allow it to cool and solidify before sealing.
8. Massage the balm into feet to relieve tiredness and promote cooling and relaxation.

Syrups and Tonics

Elderberry Immune-Boosting Syrup

Preparation Time: 10 minutes   **Cooking Time:** 45 minutes   **Servings:** Makes about 2 cups

INGREDIENTS:

- 1 cup dried elderberries
- 3 cups water
- 1 cup raw honey
- 1 cinnamon stick
- 1 teaspoon grated fresh ginger
- 1 teaspoon dried cloves

DIRECTIONS:

1. Combine the dried elderberries, water, cinnamon stick, fresh ginger, and cloves in a saucepan.
2. Bring the mixture to a boil, then reduce heat and simmer for about 45 minutes, or until the liquid is reduced by half.
3. Remove from heat and let it cool slightly.
4. Strain the mixture through a fine mesh strainer or cheesecloth into a clean bowl, pressing the berries to extract all the liquid.
5. Discard the solids and let the liquid cool to lukewarm.
6. Add the raw honey to the lukewarm liquid and stir well until fully dissolved.
7. Pour the syrup into sterilized glass bottles and store in the refrigerator.
8. To use, take 1-2 tablespoons daily for immune support, or more frequently during illness.

Ginger-Lemon Digestive Tonic

Preparation Time: 10 minutes   **Cooking Time:** 20 minutes   **Servings:** Makes about 2 cups

INGREDIENTS:

- 1 cup fresh ginger root, sliced
- 2 cups water
- 1/2 cup fresh lemon juice
- 1/2 cup raw honey

DIRECTIONS:

1. Combine the sliced ginger and water in a saucepan.
2. Bring to a boil, then reduce heat and simmer for about 20 minutes.
3. Remove from heat and let it cool slightly.
4. Strain the ginger-infused water into a clean bowl, discarding the ginger slices.
5. Add the fresh lemon juice and raw honey to the ginger-infused water, stirring well until the honey is fully dissolved.
6. Pour the tonic into sterilized glass bottles and store in the refrigerator.
7. To use, take 1-2 tablespoons before meals to aid digestion and soothe the stomach.

Chamomile-Calm Sleep Syrup

Preparation Time: 10 minutes   **Cooking Time:** 30 minutes   **Servings:** Makes about 2 cups

INGREDIENTS:

* 1 cup dried chamomile flowers
* 3 cups water
* 1 cup raw honey
* 1 teaspoon vanilla extract

DIRECTIONS:

1. Combine the dried chamomile flowers and water in a saucepan.
2. Bring the mixture to a boil, then reduce heat and simmer for about 30 minutes, or until the liquid is reduced by half.
3. Remove from heat and let it cool slightly.
4. Strain the mixture through a fine mesh strainer or cheesecloth into a clean bowl, pressing the flowers to extract all the liquid.
5. Discard the solids and let the liquid cool to lukewarm.
6. Add the raw honey and vanilla extract to the lukewarm liquid and stir well until fully dissolved.
7. Pour the syrup into sterilized glass bottles and store in the refrigerator.
8. To use, take 1-2 tablespoons before bedtime to promote relaxation and restful sleep.

Herbal Cough Syrup

Preparation Time: 10 minutes   **Cooking Time:** 30 minutes   **Servings:** Makes about 2 cups

INGREDIENTS:

* 1/2 cup dried thyme
* 1/2 cup dried mullein
* 3 cups water
* 1 cup raw honey
* 1 teaspoon fresh lemon juice

DIRECTIONS:

1. Combine the dried thyme, dried mullein, and water in a saucepan.
2. Bring the mixture to a boil, then reduce heat and simmer for about 30 minutes, or until the liquid is reduced by half.
3. Remove from heat and let it cool slightly.
4. Strain the mixture through a fine mesh strainer or cheesecloth into a clean bowl, pressing the herbs to extract all the liquid.
5. Discard the solids and let the liquid cool to lukewarm.
6. Add the raw honey and fresh lemon juice to the lukewarm liquid and stir well until fully dissolved.
7. Pour the syrup into sterilized glass bottles and store in the refrigerator.
8. To use, take 1-2 tablespoons as needed to soothe a cough and ease throat irritation.

Rosemary Memory Tonic

Preparation Time: 10 minutes   **Cooking Time:** 20 minutes   **Servings:** Makes about 2 cups

INGREDIENTS:

- 1/2 cup fresh rosemary leaves
- 2 cups water
- 1 cup raw honey
- 1 teaspoon apple cider vinegar

DIRECTIONS:

1. Combine the fresh rosemary leaves and water in a saucepan.
2. Bring to a boil, then reduce heat and simmer for about 20 minutes.
3. Remove from heat and let it cool slightly.
4. Strain the rosemary-infused water into a clean bowl, discarding the rosemary leaves.
5. Add the raw honey and apple cider vinegar to the rosemary-infused water, stirring well until the honey is fully dissolved.
6. Pour the tonic into sterilized glass bottles and store in the refrigerator.
7. To use, take 1-2 tablespoons daily to support memory and cognitive function.

CHAPTER 7

Incorporating Herbs into Your Daily Life

Cooking with Herbs: Breakfast

Herbal Oatmeal with Cinnamon and Ginger

Preparation Time: 5 minutes   **Cooking Time:** 10 minutes   **Servings:** 2

INGREDIENTS:

- 1 cup rolled oats
- 2 cups water or milk
- 1 teaspoon ground cinnamon
- 1/2 teaspoon ground ginger
- 1 tablespoon honey
- Fresh fruit (optional)

DIRECTIONS:

1. In a medium saucepan, bring water or milk to a boil.
2. Add the rolled oats, cinnamon, and ginger, stirring well.
3. Reduce heat to low and simmer for 10 minutes, stirring occasionally, until the oats are cooked and creamy.
4. Remove from heat and stir in the honey.
5. Divide the oatmeal into two bowls and top with fresh fruit if desired.
6. Serve warm and enjoy.

Nutritional Values: Calories: 210; Total Fat: 3.5g; Saturated Fat: 0.5g; Sodium: 10mg; Total Carbohydrates: 40g; Dietary Fiber: 6g; Protein: 6g; Potassium: 170mg

Chia Seed Pudding with Lavender and Blueberries

Preparation Time: 10 minutes

Cooking Time: 0 minutes
(refrigeration time: 4 hours)

Servings: 2

INGREDIENTS:

- 1/4 cup chia seeds
- 1 cup almond milk
- 1 tablespoon dried lavender flowers
- 1 tablespoon honey
- 1/2 cup fresh blueberries

DIRECTIONS:

1. In a small saucepan, gently heat the almond milk with the dried lavender flowers until warm. Do not boil.
2. Remove from heat and let it steep for 5 minutes.
3. Strain the almond milk into a bowl, discarding the lavender flowers.
4. Add the chia seeds and honey to the lavender-infused almond milk, stirring well.
5. Pour the mixture into two jars or bowls.
6. Refrigerate for at least 4 hours or overnight until the mixture thickens to a pudding-like consistency.
7. Top with fresh blueberries before serving.

Nutritional Values: Calories: 150; Total Fat: 7g; Saturated Fat: 0.5g; Sodium: 50mg; Total Carbohydrates: 19g; Dietary Fiber: 8g; Protein: 4g; Potassium: 180mg

Herbal Green Smoothie with Spinach and Mint

Preparation Time: 5 minutes

Cooking Time: 0 minutes

Servings: 2

INGREDIENTS:

- 2 cups fresh spinach
- 1/2 cup fresh mint leaves
- 1 banana
- 1 cup coconut water
- 1 tablespoon chia seeds
- 1 teaspoon honey (optional)

DIRECTIONS:

1. Place all ingredients in a blender.
2. Blend on high until smooth and creamy.
3. Taste and add honey if desired for extra sweetness.
4. Pour into two glasses and serve immediately.

Nutritional Values: Calories: 120; Total Fat: 2g; Saturated Fat: 0g; Sodium: 60mg; Total Carbohydrates: 25g; Dietary Fiber: 6g; Protein: 3g; Potassium: 470mg

Herbal Quinoa Breakfast Bowl with Turmeric and Berries

Preparation Time: 5 minutes   **Cooking Time:** 15 minutes   **Servings:** 2

INGREDIENTS:

* 1/2 cup quinoa, rinsed
* 1 cup water or milk
* 1/2 teaspoon ground turmeric
* 1 tablespoon honey
* 1/2 cup mixed berries (strawberries, blueberries, raspberries)

DIRECTIONS:

1. In a medium saucepan, bring water or milk to a boil.
2. Add the rinsed quinoa and turmeric, stirring well.
3. Reduce heat to low, cover, and simmer for 15 minutes or until the quinoa is tender and the liquid is absorbed.
4. Remove from heat and stir in the honey.
5. Divide the quinoa into two bowls and top with mixed berries.
6. Serve warm and enjoy.

Nutritional Values: Calories: 180; Total Fat: 3.5g; Saturated Fat: 0.5g; Sodium: 15mg; Total Carbohydrates: 35g; Dietary Fiber: 5g; Protein: 5g; Potassium: 260mg

Herbal Yogurt Parfait with Chamomile and Honey

Preparation Time: 10 minutes   **Cooking Time:** 0 minutes   **Servings:** 2

INGREDIENTS:

* 1 cup plain Greek yogurt
* 1 tablespoon dried chamomile flowers
* 1 tablespoon honey
* 1/2 cup granola
* 1/2 cup fresh fruit (berries, peaches, etc.)

DIRECTIONS:

1. In a small saucepan, gently heat the honey with the dried chamomile flowers until warm. Do not boil.
2. Remove from heat and let it steep for 5 minutes.
3. Strain the honey into a bowl, discarding the chamomile flowers.
4. In two serving glasses, layer the Greek yogurt, chamomile-infused honey, granola, and fresh fruit.
5. Repeat the layers until all ingredients are used.
6. Serve immediately and enjoy.

Nutritional Values: Calories: 250; Total Fat: 6g; Saturated Fat: 2g; Sodium: 60mg; Total Carbohydrates: 40g; Dietary Fiber: 5g; Protein: 12g; Potassium: 350mg

Lemon Basil Quinoa Salad

Preparation Time: 15 minutes   **Cooking Time:** 15 minutes   **Servings:** 2

INGREDIENTS:

- 1 cup quinoa, rinsed
- 2 cups water
- 1 cup cherry tomatoes, halved
- 1/2 cup cucumber, diced
- 1/4 cup fresh basil leaves, chopped
- 1/4 cup red onion, finely diced
- 1/4 cup feta cheese, crumbled
- 2 tablespoons olive oil
- 1 tablespoon fresh lemon juice
- Salt and pepper to taste

DIRECTIONS:

1. In a medium saucepan, bring the quinoa and water to a boil.
2. Reduce heat to low, cover, and simmer for 15 minutes or until the quinoa is tender and the water is absorbed.
3. Remove from heat and let it cool.
4. In a large bowl, combine the cooled quinoa, cherry tomatoes, cucumber, basil, red onion, and feta cheese.
5. In a small bowl, whisk together the olive oil, lemon juice, salt, and pepper.
6. Pour the dressing over the salad and toss gently to combine.
7. Serve immediately or refrigerate until ready to serve.

Nutritional Values: Calories: 290; Total Fat: 12g; Saturated Fat: 3g; Sodium: 220mg; Total Carbohydrates: 35g; Dietary Fiber: 5g; Protein: 10g; Potassium: 450mg

Basil Pesto Pasta Salad

Preparation Time: 15 minutes   **Cooking Time:** 10 minutes   **Servings:** 2

INGREDIENTS:

- 2 cups cooked pasta (penne or fusilli)
- 1/2 cup cherry tomatoes, halved
- 1/4 cup black olives, sliced
- 1/4 cup fresh basil pesto
- 1/4 cup fresh basil leaves, chopped
- 2 tablespoons pine nuts, toasted
- 1/4 cup grated Parmesan cheese
- Salt and pepper to taste

DIRECTIONS:

1. Cook the pasta according to the package instructions, then drain and let cool.
2. In a large bowl, combine the cooked pasta, cherry tomatoes, black olives, and fresh basil pesto.
3. Toss gently to coat the pasta with the pesto.
4. Add the chopped basil leaves, toasted pine nuts, and grated Parmesan cheese.
5. Season with salt and pepper to taste.
6. Serve immediately or refrigerate until ready to serve.

Nutritional Values: Calories: 400; Total Fat: 20g; Saturated Fat: 4g; Sodium: 320mg; Total Carbohydrates: 45g; Dietary Fiber: 3g; Protein: 12g; Potassium: 350mg

Thyme and Lemon Baked Salmon

Preparation Time: 10 minutes   **Cooking Time:** 20 minutes   **Servings:** 2

INGREDIENTS:

- 2 salmon fillets
- 1 tablespoon fresh thyme, chopped
- 1 tablespoon olive oil
- 1 tablespoon fresh lemon juice
- Salt and pepper to taste
- Lemon slices for garnish

DIRECTIONS:

1. Preheat the oven to 375°F (190°C).
2. Place the salmon fillets on a baking sheet lined with parchment paper.
3. In a small bowl, mix the chopped thyme, olive oil, lemon juice, salt, and pepper.
4. Brush the thyme and lemon mixture over the salmon fillets.
5. Bake for 20 minutes or until the salmon is cooked through and flakes easily with a fork.
6. Garnish with lemon slices and serve with a side of vegetables or salad.

Nutritional Values: Calories: 280; Total Fat: 16g; Saturated Fat: 3g; Sodium: 60mg; Total Carbohydrates: 1g; Dietary Fiber: 0g; Protein: 30g; Potassium: 600mg

Rosemary Chicken Wraps

Preparation Time: 10 minutes   **Cooking Time:** 15 minutes   **Servings:** 2

INGREDIENTS:

- 2 boneless, skinless chicken breasts
- 1 tablespoon fresh rosemary, chopped
- 1 tablespoon olive oil
- Salt and pepper to taste
- 2 whole wheat tortillas
- 1/2 cup mixed greens
- 1/4 cup shredded carrots
- 1/4 cup cucumber, sliced
- 2 tablespoons hummus

DIRECTIONS:

1. Season the chicken breasts with rosemary, olive oil, salt, and pepper.
2. Heat a grill pan over medium-high heat and cook the chicken for 6-7 minutes on each side, or until fully cooked.
3. Let the chicken rest for a few minutes, then slice thinly.
4. Warm the tortillas in a dry skillet over medium heat.
5. Spread hummus evenly on each tortilla.
6. Top with mixed greens, shredded carrots, cucumber slices, and sliced chicken.
7. Roll up the tortillas, slice in half, and serve immediately.

Nutritional Values: Calories: 350; Total Fat: 14g; Saturated Fat: 2g; Sodium: 400mg; Total Carbohydrates: 30g; Dietary Fiber: 6g; Protein: 30g; Potassium: 600mg

Mint and Pea Soup

Preparation Time: 10 minutes   **Cooking Time:** 20 minutes   **Servings:** 2

INGREDIENTS:

- 2 cups fresh or frozen peas
- 1 small onion, chopped
- 2 cups vegetable broth
- 1/4 cup fresh mint leaves, chopped
- 1/2 cup plain yogurt
- 1 tablespoon olive oil
- Salt and pepper to taste

DIRECTIONS:

1. Heat olive oil in a large pot over medium heat.
2. Add the chopped onion and cook until softened, about 5 minutes.
3. Add the peas and vegetable broth, bringing to a boil.
4. Reduce heat and simmer for 10 minutes, until the peas are tender.
5. Remove from heat and stir in the fresh mint leaves.
6. Use an immersion blender to puree the soup until smooth.
7. Stir in the yogurt, season with salt and pepper, and serve warm.

Nutritional Values: Calories: 200; Total Fat: 8g; Saturated Fat: 1.5g; Sodium: 450mg; Total Carbohydrates: 25g; Dietary Fiber: 8g; Protein: 9g; Potassium: 500mg

Sage and Lemon Chicken

Preparation Time: 10 minutes   **Cooking Time:** 25 minutes   **Servings:** 2

INGREDIENTS:

- 2 boneless, skinless chicken breasts
- 1 tablespoon fresh sage, chopped
- 1 tablespoon olive oil
- 1 tablespoon fresh lemon juice
- Salt and pepper to taste
- Lemon slices for garnish

DIRECTIONS:

1. Preheat the oven to 375°F (190°C).
2. In a small bowl, mix the chopped sage, olive oil, lemon juice, salt, and pepper.
3. Rub the mixture over the chicken breasts.
4. Place the chicken breasts in a baking dish and bake for 25 minutes, or until the chicken is cooked through and no longer pink in the center.
5. Garnish with lemon slices and serve with a side of vegetables or a salad.

Nutritional Values: Calories: 280; Total Fat: 12g; Saturated Fat: 2g; Sodium: 70mg; Total Carbohydrates: 2g; Dietary Fiber: 1g; Protein: 36g; Potassium: 450mg

Rosemary Roasted Vegetables

Preparation Time: 10 minutes | **Cooking Time:** 30 minutes | **Servings:** 2

INGREDIENTS:

- 1 cup baby carrots
- 1 cup Brussels sprouts, halved
- 1 cup butternut squash, cubed
- 1 tablespoon fresh rosemary, chopped
- 2 tablespoons olive oil
- Salt and pepper to taste

DIRECTIONS:

1. Preheat the oven to 400°F (200°C).
2. In a large bowl, combine the baby carrots, Brussels sprouts, butternut squash, rosemary, olive oil, salt, and pepper.
3. Toss the vegetables to coat them evenly with the oil and seasoning.
4. Spread the vegetables on a baking sheet in a single layer.
5. Roast for 30 minutes, or until the vegetables are tender and lightly browned.
6. Serve warm as a side dish or over a bed of greens.

Nutritional Values: Calories: 180; Total Fat: 10g; Saturated Fat: 1.5g; Sodium: 100mg; Total Carbohydrates: 22g; Dietary Fiber: 6g; Protein: 3g; Potassium: 600mg

Turmeric and Ginger Lentil Soup

Preparation Time: 10 minutes | **Cooking Time:** 30 minutes | **Servings:** 2

INGREDIENTS:

- 1 cup red lentils, rinsed
- 1 small onion, chopped
- 2 cloves garlic, minced
- 1 tablespoon fresh ginger, grated
- 1 teaspoon ground turmeric
- 4 cups vegetable broth
- 1 tablespoon olive oil
- Salt and pepper to taste
- Fresh cilantro for garnish (optional)

DIRECTIONS:

1. Heat olive oil in a large pot over medium heat.
2. Add the chopped onion and cook until softened, about 5 minutes.
3. Add the garlic, ginger, and turmeric, and cook for another minute.
4. Add the red lentils and vegetable broth, bringing the mixture to a boil.
5. Reduce heat and simmer for 30 minutes, or until the lentils are tender.
6. Season with salt and pepper to taste.
7. Garnish with fresh cilantro if desired, and serve warm.

Nutritional Values: Calories: 250; Total Fat: 7g; Saturated Fat: 1g; Sodium: 400mg; Total Carbohydrates: 35g; Dietary Fiber: 12g; Protein: 14g; Potassium: 600mg

Thyme and Garlic Baked Cod

Preparation Time: 10 minutes   **Cooking Time:** 20 minutes   **Servings:** 2

INGREDIENTS:

- 2 cod fillets
- 2 cloves garlic, minced
- 1 tablespoon fresh thyme, chopped
- 2 tablespoons olive oil
- Salt and pepper to taste
- Lemon wedges for serving

DIRECTIONS:

1. Preheat the oven to 375°F (190°C).
2. In a small bowl, mix the minced garlic, chopped thyme, olive oil, salt, and pepper.
3. Rub the mixture over the cod fillets.
4. Place the cod fillets in a baking dish and bake for 20 minutes, or until the fish is opaque and flakes easily with a fork.
5. Serve with lemon wedges and a side of vegetables or rice.

Nutritional Values: Calories: 220; Total Fat: 11g; Saturated Fat: 2g; Sodium: 90mg; Total Carbohydrates: 1g; Dietary Fiber: 0g; Protein: 28g; Potassium: 450mg

Basil and Tomato Stuffed Peppers

Preparation Time: 15 minutes   **Cooking Time:** 30 minutes   **Servings:** 2

INGREDIENTS:

- 2 large bell peppers, halved and seeded
- 1 cup cooked quinoa
- 1 cup cherry tomatoes, halved
- 1/4 cup fresh basil leaves, chopped
- 1/4 cup grated Parmesan cheese
- 1 tablespoon olive oil
- Salt and pepper to taste

DIRECTIONS:

1. Preheat the oven to 375°F (190°C).
2. In a large bowl, combine the cooked quinoa, cherry tomatoes, basil leaves, Parmesan cheese, olive oil, salt, and pepper.
3. Stuff the bell pepper halves with the quinoa mixture.
4. Place the stuffed peppers in a baking dish and cover with foil.
5. Bake for 30 minutes, or until the peppers are tender.
6. Remove the foil and bake for an additional 5 minutes to lightly brown the tops.
7. Serve warm as a main dish or side.

Nutritional Values: Calories: 280; Total Fat: 12g; Saturated Fat: 3g; Sodium: 220mg; Total Carbohydrates: 35g; Dietary Fiber: 7g; Protein: 10g; Potassium: 600mg

Berry and Lavender Smoothie

Preparation Time: 5 minutes   **Cooking Time:** 0 minutes   **Servings:** 2

INGREDIENTS:

- 1 cup mixed berries (strawberries, blueberries, raspberries)
- 1 banana
- 1/2 cup Greek yogurt
- 1/2 teaspoon dried lavender flowers
- 1 tablespoon honey
- 1 cup almond milk

DIRECTIONS:

1. Place the mixed berries, banana, Greek yogurt, dried lavender flowers, honey, and almond milk in a blender.
2. Blend on high until smooth and creamy.
3. Pour into two glasses and serve immediately.

Nutritional Values: Calories: 210; Total Fat: 4g; Saturated Fat: 1.5g; Sodium: 50mg; Total Carbohydrates: 40g; Dietary Fiber: 6g; Protein: 8g; Potassium: 500mg

Chamomile and Peach Smoothie

Preparation Time: 5 minutes   **Cooking Time:** 0 minutes   **Servings:** 2

INGREDIENTS:

- 2 ripe peaches, peeled and sliced
- 1 banana
- 1/2 cup Greek yogurt
- 1/2 cup brewed chamomile tea, cooled
- 1 tablespoon honey
- 1/2 teaspoon vanilla extract

DIRECTIONS:

1. Place the peaches, banana, Greek yogurt, cooled chamomile tea, honey, and vanilla extract in a blender.
2. Blend on high until smooth and creamy.
3. Pour into two glasses and serve immediately.

Nutritional Values: Calories: 190; Total Fat: 3g; Saturated Fat: 1.5g; Sodium: 40mg; Total Carbohydrates: 40g; Dietary Fiber: 4g; Protein: 6g; Potassium: 500mg

Ginger and Turmeric Immunity Juice

Preparation Time: 5 minutes   **Cooking Time:** 0 minutes   **Servings:** 2

INGREDIENTS:

* 1 large carrot, peeled and chopped
* 1 apple, cored and chopped
* 1 orange, peeled and segmented
* 1-inch piece fresh ginger, peeled
* 1/2 teaspoon ground turmeric
* 1 cup water

DIRECTIONS:

1. Place the carrot, apple, orange, ginger, turmeric, and water in a blender.
2. Blend on high until smooth.
3. Strain the juice through a fine mesh strainer into two glasses, pressing the pulp to extract all the liquid.
4. Serve immediately.

Nutritional Values: Calories: 120; Total Fat: 0.5g; Saturated Fat: 0g; Sodium: 10mg; Total Carbohydrates: 30g; Dietary Fiber: 6g; Protein: 1g; Potassium: 450mg

Mint and Cucumber Refreshing Smoothie

Preparation Time: 5 minutes   **Cooking Time:** 0 minutes   **Servings:** 2

INGREDIENTS:

* 1 cucumber, peeled and chopped
* 1/2 cup fresh mint leaves
* 1 green apple, cored and chopped
* 1 tablespoon fresh lime juice
* 1 cup cold water

DIRECTIONS:

1. Place the cucumber, mint leaves, green apple, lime juice, and cold water in a blender.
2. Blend on high until smooth.
3. Pour into two glasses and serve immediately.

Nutritional Values: Calories: 60; Total Fat: 0g; Saturated Fat: 0g; Sodium: 10mg; Total Carbohydrates: 15g; Dietary Fiber: 4g; Protein: 1g; Potassium: 280mg

Green Detox Smoothie with Spirulina

Preparation Time: 5 minutes   **Cooking Time:** 0 minutes   **Servings:** 2

INGREDIENTS:

- 1 cup spinach
- 1/2 cup kale
- 1 banana
- 1/2 cup pineapple chunks
- 1 teaspoon spirulina powder
- 1 tablespoon chia seeds
- 1 cup coconut water

DIRECTIONS:

1. Place all ingredients in a blender.
2. Blend on high until smooth and creamy.
3. Pour into two glasses and serve immediately.

Nutritional Values: Calories: 180; Total Fat: 3g; Saturated Fat: 1g; Sodium: 45mg; Total Carbohydrates: 35g; Dietary Fiber: 8g; Protein: 5g; Potassium: 720mg

Herbal Self-Care Practices: Bath Soaks and Body Scrubs

Lavender Epsom Salt Bath Soak

Preparation Time: 5 minutes   **Cooking Time:** 0 minutes   **Servings:** 2

INGREDIENTS:

- 2 cups Epsom salt
- 1/2 cup dried lavender flowers
- 10 drops lavender essential oil
- 1/4 cup baking soda

DIRECTIONS:

1. In a large mixing bowl, combine the Epsom salt, dried lavender flowers, and baking soda.
2. Add the lavender essential oil and mix thoroughly.
3. Transfer the mixture to a clean, airtight container.
4. To use, add 1 cup of the mixture to warm bathwater and stir to dissolve.
5. Soak in the bath for at least 20 minutes to relax muscles and calm the mind.

Rosemary and Mint Foot Soak

Preparation Time: 5 minutes   **Cooking Time:** 10 minutes   **Servings:** 2

INGREDIENTS:

- 1/2 cup fresh rosemary leaves
- 1/2 cup fresh mint leaves
- 2 cups Epsom salt
- 1/4 cup baking soda

DIRECTIONS:

1. Bring 4 cups of water to a boil in a large pot.
2. Add the fresh rosemary and mint leaves, and let it simmer for 10 minutes.
3. Remove from heat and strain the herbs, reserving the infused water.
4. In a large basin, combine the Epsom salt and baking soda.
5. Pour the infused water over the salt mixture and stir to dissolve.
6. Soak your feet in the mixture for 15-20 minutes to relieve tired, aching feet.

Chamomile and Oatmeal Body Scrub

Preparation Time: 10 minutes   **Cooking Time:** 0 minutes   **Servings:** 2

INGREDIENTS:

- 1 cup rolled oats
- 1/2 cup dried chamomile flowers
- 1/2 cup coconut oil, melted
- 1/4 cup brown sugar
- 10 drops chamomile essential oil

DIRECTIONS:

1. In a food processor, pulse the rolled oats and dried chamomile flowers until they are finely ground.
2. In a large mixing bowl, combine the ground oats and chamomile with the brown sugar.
3. Add the melted coconut oil and chamomile essential oil, mixing thoroughly.
4. Transfer the scrub to a clean, airtight container.
5. To use, apply a generous amount to damp skin in the shower or bath, gently massaging in circular motions. Rinse off with warm water.

Lemon and Rosemary Sugar Scrub

Preparation Time: 10 minutes   **Cooking Time:** 0 minutes   **Servings:** 2

INGREDIENTS:

- 1 cup granulated sugar
- 1/2 cup coconut oil, melted
- 2 tablespoons fresh rosemary, finely chopped
- Zest of 1 lemon
- 10 drops lemon essential oil

DIRECTIONS:

1. In a large mixing bowl, combine the granulated sugar, chopped rosemary, and lemon zest.
2. Add the melted coconut oil and lemon essential oil, mixing thoroughly.
3. Transfer the scrub to a clean, airtight container.
4. To use, apply a generous amount to damp skin in the shower, gently massaging in circular motions. Rinse off with warm water.

Calendula and Honey Bath Soak

Preparation Time: 5 minutes | **Cooking Time:** 0 minutes | **Servings:** 2

INGREDIENTS:

- 1 cup dried calendula flowers
- 2 cups Epsom salt
- 1/4 cup honey
- 10 drops chamomile essential oil

DIRECTIONS:

1. In a large mixing bowl, combine the Epsom salt and dried calendula flowers.
2. Add the honey and chamomile essential oil, mixing thoroughly.
3. Transfer the mixture to a clean, airtight container.
4. To use, add 1 cup of the mixture to warm bathwater and stir to dissolve.
5. Soak in the bath for at least 20 minutes to soothe and nourish the skin.

Herbal Self-Care Practices: Aromatherapy and Essential Oils

Aromatherapy and essential oils have been integral to holistic health practices for centuries. This therapeutic practice involves using aromatic plant extracts and essential oils to enhance physical and psychological well-being. The use of essential oils in aromatherapy taps into the profound connection between the sense of smell and the brain, particularly the limbic system, which is responsible for emotions, memories, and arousal. This connection is why specific scents can evoke powerful emotional responses and memories.

Obtaining essential oils requires a number of different procedures, including steam distillation, cold pressing, and solvent extraction, among others. Essential oils are highly concentrated plant extracts. Essential oils are comprised of a variety of different chemicals, each of which possesses a unique set of medicinal characteristics. As an illustration, lavender oil is well-known for its ability to induce feelings of tranquility and relaxation, whereas peppermint oil is exhilarating and has the potential to improve alertness and concentration. Due to their adaptability, essential oils are extremely useful instruments that can be utilized in a variety of therapeutic applications, including those that are more specific in nature.

One of the primary methods of using essential oils in aromatherapy is through inhalation. This can be achieved by using diffusers, which disperse the oils into the air, allowing the aromatic compounds to be inhaled and absorbed through the respiratory system. Another method is the steam inhalation technique, where a few drops of essential oil are added to a bowl of hot water, and the individual inhales the steam, often with a towel draped over the head to create a tent-like effect. Inhalation is particularly effective for respiratory issues, emotional well-being, and stress relief.

Topical application is another common use of essential oils, where the oils are absorbed through the skin. It is essential to dilute essential oils with a carrier oil, such as jojoba, almond, or coconut oil, to avoid skin irritation and ensure safe application. For instance, a blend of lavender and chamomile oils diluted in a carrier oil can be massaged into the skin to promote relaxation and sleep. Similarly, eucalyptus or tea tree oil, when diluted, can be applied to the chest or back to alleviate symptoms of colds and respiratory infections.

Aromatherapy can also be incorporated into various self-care practices. Adding essential oils to bathwater creates a luxurious and therapeutic experience. For example, adding a few drops of lavender or rose oil to a warm bath can help relax the body and mind, providing a perfect end to a stressful day. Similarly, essential oils can be added to body lotions, scrubs, or even homemade cleaning products to infuse their therapeutic properties into daily routines.

The therapeutic effects of essential oils are supported by a growing body of scientific research. Studies have shown that lavender oil can significantly reduce anxiety and improve sleep quality. In a study conducted by the University of Miami, participants who inhaled lavender oil experienced decreased anxiety, improved mood, and enhanced cognitive performance. Similarly, research on peppermint oil has demonstrated its efficacy in improving alertness and cognitive performance, making it an excellent choice for combating mental fatigue and enhancing focus.

Real-world examples of aromatherapy's benefits are plentiful. Many hospitals and clinics now incorporate essential oils into patient care to reduce stress and anxiety. For instance, lavender and peppermint oils are often used in oncology units to help patients manage nausea and anxiety associated with chemotherapy. Additionally, essential oils are widely used in massage therapy to enhance the therapeutic benefits of the treatment, providing both physical and emotional relief.

When using essential oils, it is crucial to consider safety and quality. Not all essential oils are created equal, and the purity and quality of the oils can significantly impact their effectiveness and safety. It is advisable to purchase oils from reputable suppliers who provide detailed information about their sourcing and production methods. Additionally, some essential oils can interact with medications or may not be suitable for individuals with certain health conditions, so it is essential to consult with a healthcare provider or a certified aromatherapist when incorporating new oils into a health regimen.

Herbal Self-Care Practices: Meditation and Relaxation Techniques

Meditation and relaxation techniques have long been recognized as integral components of holistic health practices, providing profound benefits for both the mind and body. These practices, rooted in ancient traditions, have been scientifically validated for their efficacy in reducing stress, enhancing emotional well-being, and promoting overall health. Incorporating herbs into these techniques can further amplify their effects, creating a synergistic approach to achieving tranquility and balance.

At its foundation, meditation is a practice that entails training the mind to achieve a state of concentrated attention and heightened awareness throughout the practice. A number of different types of meditation, including mindfulness meditation, transcendental meditation, and guided visualization, each have their own set of advantages and may be adapted to meet the specific requirements of each individual. Meditation that focuses on mindfulness, for example, places an emphasis on being aware of the present moment and observing thoughts and feelings without passing judgment on them. It has been demonstrated that engaging in this technique can alleviate symptoms of anxiety and depression, bring about improvements in cognitive performance, and strengthen emotional regulation.

Integrating herbal remedies into meditation practices can enhance their effectiveness. Herbs such as lavender, chamomile, and lemon balm are renowned for their calming properties and can be used in various forms, such as teas, tinctures, or essential oils, to facilitate relaxation and mental clarity. For example, drinking a cup of chamomile tea before a meditation session can help to calm the nervous system and prepare the mind for deep focus. Similarly, diffusing lavender essential oil in the meditation space can create a serene environment conducive to relaxation.

Relaxation techniques, including progressive muscle relaxation, deep breathing exercises, and yoga, also play a vital role in managing stress and promoting well-being. Progressive muscle relaxation involves systematically tensing and relaxing different muscle groups, helping to release physical tension and increase body awareness. This technique can be particularly effective when combined with the use of herbal oils. For instance, massaging the muscles with a blend of lavender and peppermint oils can enhance the relaxation response and provide additional relief from tension.

Deep breathing exercises, such as diaphragmatic breathing and the 4-7-8 breathing technique, are powerful tools for activating the body's relaxation response. These exercises help to slow the heart rate, lower blood pressure, and reduce levels of the stress hormone cortisol. Incorporating aromatherapy into these practices can further enhance their benefits. Inhaling the scent of calming herbs like valerian root or passionflower during deep breathing exercises can help to deepen relaxation and improve the overall efficacy of the practice.

Another highly efficient method of relaxation is yoga, which is a practice that blends physical postures, the regulation of one's breath, and meditation. Certain yoga poses, such as the Child's Pose (Balasana) and the Legs-Up-The-Wall Pose (Viparita Karani), are very helpful for reducing stress and bringing about a state of calm. The use of herbal teas, essential oils, or even herbal compresses are all viable options for incorporating herbal medicines into a yoga regimen. There are also more options available. A calming herbal tea, such as lemon balm, can be consumed prior to a yoga session in order to boost the calming effects of the practice. Additionally, using a herbal compress to muscles that are experiencing pain can assist in the recuperation process and promote relaxation.

Real-world examples of the successful integration of herbs into meditation and relaxation practices abound. Many wellness centers and spas incorporate herbal remedies into their relaxation therapies.

For instance, herbal steam rooms use the vapors of eucalyptus, peppermint, and other herbs to promote respiratory health and relaxation. Similarly, herbal massage oils infused with calming herbs are commonly used in therapeutic massage to enhance relaxation and relieve muscle tension.

Research supports the benefits of combining herbs with meditation and relaxation techniques. Studies have shown that the use of lavender essential oil can significantly reduce anxiety and improve mood. A study published in the "Journal of Clinical Psychopharmacology" found that lavender oil was as effective as lorazepam, a common anti-anxiety medication, in reducing anxiety symptoms. Similarly, research on chamomile has demonstrated its efficacy in promoting relaxation and improving sleep quality.

Meditation and relaxation techniques are essential tools for managing stress and enhancing overall well-being. The incorporation of herbal remedies into these practices can further amplify their benefits, creating a holistic approach to achieving tranquility and balance. Whether through the use of calming teas, aromatic essential oils, or soothing herbal compresses, herbs can play a significant role in enhancing the effectiveness of meditation and relaxation techniques. By integrating these practices into daily life, individuals can harness the power of nature to support mental and physical health, fostering a deeper sense of peace and well-being.

CHAPTER 8
Advanced Herbal Techniques and Applications

8.1 Creating Custom Herbal Blends

The process of creating individualized herbal mixtures is both an art and a science, and it enables individuals to personalize herbal medicines to their particular health requirements and preferences. The practice of combining various herbs in order to produce a synergistic impact, in which the combined action of the herbs is higher than the sum of their separate effects, is referred to as the synergistic effect. Creating bespoke mixtures calls for an in-depth knowledge of the characteristics of a wide range of herbs, the ways in which they interact with one another, and the most effective ways in which they can be applied to address particular health concerns.

The process of creating custom herbal blends begins with identifying the desired outcome or therapeutic goal. This could range from enhancing immunity, improving digestion, alleviating stress, or promoting sleep. Once the objective is clear, the next step is to select herbs that are known to support these specific functions. For instance, if the goal is to create a blend for stress relief, herbs such as lavender, chamomile, and lemon balm, known for their calming properties, would be ideal choices.

Understanding the energetic properties of herbs is also crucial in creating effective blends. In traditional herbal medicine, herbs are often classified according to their energetic qualities, such as warming, cooling, drying, or moistening effects. This classification helps in balancing the blend to match the individual's constitution and the nature of their condition. For example, someone with a cold and damp constitution might benefit from warming and drying herbs like ginger and cinnamon, while someone with a hot and dry constitution might find cooling and moistening herbs like peppermint and marshmallow root more beneficial.

Proportion and synergy are key elements in crafting custom blends. It's essential to balance the proportions of the herbs to ensure that the blend is both effective and palatable. Typically, a blend consists of a primary herb (the main herb that addresses the primary concern), secondary herbs (supporting herbs that enhance the primary herb's action), and adjunctive herbs (herbs that address secondary symptoms or improve the blend's taste). For instance, in a blend aimed at supporting sleep, valerian root might be the primary herb due to its strong sedative properties, while secondary herbs like passionflower and hops enhance the overall calming effect, and adjunctive herbs like peppermint improve the flavor.

When creating a custom blend, it's also important to consider the form in which the herbs will be consumed. Herbal teas, tinctures, capsules, and topical applications all have different preparation methods and absorption rates. Teas and tinctures are often preferred for their rapid absorption and ease of preparation. For instance, a calming tea blend might include equal parts of chamomile, lemon balm, and passionflower, brewed for 10-15 minutes to extract the active compounds. In contrast, a tincture blend for digestive support might combine ginger, fennel, and peppermint, with the herbs soaked in alcohol for several weeks to create a potent extract.

Real-world examples of successful custom herbal blends can provide valuable insights. Consider the case of a client with chronic anxiety who experiences difficulty sleeping. A custom blend might include valerian root and passionflower for their sedative effects, combined with lavender to reduce anxiety and peppermint to aid digestion and improve the blend's flavor. By adjusting the proportions based on the client's response, a personalized remedy can be created that effectively addresses both the anxiety and sleep issues.

Creating custom herbal blends also involves a process of experimentation and adjustment. Each individual's response to herbs can vary, and it may take some time to find the perfect combination and dosage. Keeping detailed notes on the herbs used, proportions, and the individual's response can help refine the blend over time. This iterative process ensures that the final product is both effective and well-tolerated.

Safety considerations are paramount when creating custom blends. It's essential to be aware of any potential herb-drug interactions, contraindications, and the overall safety profile of each herb. Consulting reliable sources and, if necessary, seeking guidance from a qualified herbalist or healthcare provider can prevent adverse effects and ensure the blend's safety and efficacy.

8.2 Herbal Fermentation and Preservation Methods

Herbal fermentation and preservation methods are crucial techniques in the field of herbal medicine, ensuring the longevity and potency of medicinal herbs. These methods not only extend the shelf life of herbs but also can enhance their therapeutic properties through the fermentation process. By understanding and applying these techniques, herbalists can create potent, stable, and effective remedies that maintain their efficacy over time.

Fermentation is an age-old practice that involves the transformation of herbs through the action of microorganisms such as bacteria, yeast, and fungi. This process not only preserves the herbs but also often enhances their bioavailability and therapeutic effects. For example, fermented herbs can produce beneficial compounds such as probiotics, enzymes, and organic acids, which can enhance gut health, improve digestion, and boost the immune system.

One of the most common methods of herbal fermentation is lacto-fermentation, which uses lactic acid bacteria to ferment the herbs. This method is widely used in the preparation of fermented foods and beverages, such as kimchi, sauerkraut, and kombucha. Lacto-fermented herbal remedies can be made by mixing fresh or dried herbs with salt and water, allowing the mixture to ferment in a controlled environment. For instance, a simple recipe for fermented garlic involves peeling and crushing fresh garlic cloves, placing them in a jar, and covering them with a brine solution made of water and salt. The jar is then sealed and left at room temperature for several days to weeks, depending on the desired level of fermentation. The result is a tangy, probiotic-rich garlic that retains its medicinal properties and has an enhanced flavor.

Another method of herbal fermentation involves the use of kombucha, a fermented tea made with a symbiotic culture of bacteria and yeast (SCOBY). Herbs can be added to the kombucha during the fermentation process to create a medicinal beverage. For example, adding ginger and turmeric to kombucha can produce a powerful anti-inflammatory drink. The herbs infuse the kombucha with their medicinal properties, while the fermentation process increases the bioavailability of the active compounds.

Preservation methods for herbs are equally important in maintaining their therapeutic efficacy. Drying is one of the oldest and simplest methods of preserving herbs. By removing moisture, drying prevents the growth of mold and bacteria, thereby extending the shelf life of the herbs. There are several drying methods, including air drying, oven drying, and using a dehydrator. Air drying is suitable for herbs with low moisture content, such as rosemary, thyme, and oregano. These herbs can be tied into small bundles and hung upside down in a well-ventilated, dark, and dry area. Oven drying and dehydrators are more suitable for herbs with higher moisture content, such as basil, mint, and tarragon. These methods require careful monitoring to avoid overheating, which can degrade the essential oils and reduce the potency of the herbs.

Freezing is another effective preservation method, particularly for herbs that do not dry well, such as chives, cilantro, and parsley. Herbs can be frozen in various forms, such as whole leaves, chopped, or as herb-infused ice cubes. To freeze herbs, they should be washed, patted dry, and spread out on a baking sheet to freeze individually before being transferred to airtight containers or freezer bags. Herb-infused ice cubes can be made by chopping the herbs, placing them in ice cube trays, and covering them with water or olive oil before freezing. These herb cubes can be conveniently added to soups, stews, and sauces.

Tinctures are another excellent method of preserving the medicinal properties of herbs. A tincture is a concentrated liquid extract made by soaking herbs in alcohol or vinegar. The alcohol acts as a solvent, extracting the active compounds from the herbs and preserving them for extended periods. Tinctures can be made with fresh or dried herbs, with a typical ratio being one part herb to four parts alcohol for fresh herbs, and one part herb to five parts alcohol for dried herbs. The mixture is stored in a dark, cool place for several weeks, shaken daily to aid the extraction process, and then strained to remove the plant material. The resulting tincture can be stored in dark glass bottles and used as needed, with a typical dosage being one to two droppers full diluted in water or juice.

Vinegar infusions and herbal oils are two more methods that are helpful in preserving herbs, in addition to the ones described above. As with the preparation of a tincture, the process of preparing a vinegar infusion involves soaking herbs in vinegar. However, instead of utilizing alcohol, vinegar is used. This technique is especially well-suited for culinary herbs like rosemary, thyme, and sage, and it may be utilized to produce herbal vinegars that are both tasty and medicinal in nature. Infusing herbs into carrier oils, such as olive oil, coconut oil, or almond oil, is the process that results in the production of herbal oils. This technique is frequently utilized in the production of herbal massage oils, salves, and balms. The herbs are steeped in the carrier oil for a number of weeks, often in a warm atmosphere, and then they are strained after the process is complete. The herbal oil that is produced can be applied topically to treat a variety of skin diseases and can also be utilized for massage therapy.

Real-world examples of herbal fermentation and preservation methods highlight their practical applications. For instance, in traditional Korean medicine, fermented herbal preparations are used extensively to enhance the potency of medicinal herbs. Similarly, in Ayurvedic medicine, certain herbs are fermented to increase their efficacy and reduce potential side effects.

8.3 Integrating Herbal Remedies with Conventional Medicine

Integrating herbal remedies with conventional medicine represents a holistic approach to healthcare, merging the time-tested wisdom of natural medicine with the advancements of modern medical science. This integration can offer comprehensive treatment options that address the root causes of health issues while managing symptoms effectively. However, it requires careful consideration, knowledge, and collaboration between healthcare providers and patients to ensure safety and efficacy.

The rationale behind integrating herbal remedies with conventional medicine lies in the complementary benefits they can provide. Herbal remedies often offer fewer side effects compared to synthetic pharmaceuticals, making them suitable for long-term use in chronic conditions. Additionally, herbs can support the body's natural healing processes, improve overall wellness, and prevent disease, while conventional medicine can provide targeted, rapid interventions for acute conditions.

One of the primary considerations when integrating herbal remedies with conventional medicine is understanding potential herb-drug interactions. Herbs can interact with pharmaceuticals in various ways, such as altering drug metabolism, enhancing or diminishing drug effects, and impacting drug absorption. For example, St. John's Wort, a popular herb used for depression, can induce liver enzymes that metabolize drugs, potentially reducing the effectiveness of medications like birth control pills and certain antidepressants. Therefore, it is crucial for patients to inform their healthcare providers about all the herbs and supplements they are taking to avoid adverse interactions and ensure coordinated care.

A successful integration strategy involves a thorough evaluation of the patient's overall health, medical history, and current treatments. This holistic assessment allows healthcare providers to recommend appropriate herbal remedies that complement conventional treatments. For instance, a patient undergoing chemotherapy for cancer might benefit from ginger or peppermint to alleviate nausea, or from ginseng to boost energy levels and support immune function. Such integrative approaches can improve the patient's quality of life and potentially enhance treatment outcomes.

Real-world examples illustrate the potential benefits of integrating herbal remedies with conventional medicine. In oncology, integrative oncology centers incorporate herbal medicine to support patients through their cancer treatments. Herbs such as turmeric, with its anti-inflammatory and antioxidant properties, are used alongside conventional treatments to help manage inflammation and oxidative stress. Similarly, milk thistle is often recommended to support liver function in patients taking hepatotoxic medications.

In cardiovascular health, hawthorn has been used to complement conventional treatments for heart failure and hypertension. Studies have shown that hawthorn can improve heart function, increase exercise tolerance, and reduce symptoms such as fatigue and shortness of breath. Integrating hawthorn with standard heart medications, under the guidance of a healthcare provider, can provide a balanced approach to managing cardiovascular conditions.

Another area where herbal remedies can complement conventional medicine is in managing chronic pain. Turmeric, ginger, and willow bark are herbs known for their anti-inflammatory and analgesic properties. These herbs can be used alongside conventional pain medications to reduce inflammation and pain, potentially allowing for lower doses of pharmaceuticals and reducing the risk of side effects.

To facilitate the safe and effective integration of herbal remedies with conventional medicine, education and communication are essential. Healthcare providers need to stay informed about the latest research on herbal medicine, understand the pharmacology of herbs, and be aware of potential interactions with drugs. Patients should feel empowered to discuss their use of herbal remedies openly with their healthcare providers, ensuring that all aspects of their treatment plan are considered.

Integrative health clinics and practitioners play a crucial role in this process. These professionals are trained in both conventional and herbal medicine, providing a bridge between the two approaches. They can develop comprehensive treatment plans that incorporate herbal remedies, nutritional support, lifestyle modifications, and conventional therapies tailored to the individual needs of the patient.

Moreover, clinical research and trials are increasingly focusing on the integration of herbal medicine with conventional treatments. These studies are essential for validating the efficacy and safety of herbal remedies, understanding their mechanisms of action, and identifying optimal dosages and formulations. Evidence-based practice is the cornerstone of integrative medicine, ensuring that recommendations are supported by scientific research.

In practice, integrating herbal remedies with conventional medicine often involves the following steps:

- **Assessment:** Conduct a comprehensive health assessment, including medical history, current medications, lifestyle, and dietary habits.
- **Education:** Educate patients about the benefits and risks of herbal remedies, potential interactions with medications, and the importance of informed consent.
- **Collaboration:** Work collaboratively with other healthcare providers, including doctors, pharmacists, and integrative health practitioners, to develop a coordinated treatment plan.
- **Monitoring:** Regularly monitor the patient's response to treatment, adjusting the herbal and conventional therapies as needed to achieve the best outcomes.
- **Documentation:** Keep detailed records of all treatments, including herbal remedies, to track progress and make informed decisions.

Integrating herbal remedies with conventional medicine offers a comprehensive approach to healthcare that leverages the strengths of both systems. This integrative approach can enhance patient outcomes, improve quality of life, and provide more holistic care. However, it requires careful consideration of potential interactions, ongoing education, and open communication between patients and healthcare providers. By fostering a collaborative and informed environment, the integration of herbal and conventional medicine can be both safe and highly effective, paving the way for a more holistic and patient-centered approach to health and wellness.

8.4 Case Studies: Real-Life Success Stories

The integration of herbal remedies into conventional medicine has produced numerous real-life success stories that highlight the potential benefits of this holistic approach. These case studies demonstrate how personalized herbal treatments can complement standard medical practices, leading to improved patient outcomes and enhanced quality of life.

Case Study 1: Managing Chronic Pain with Herbal Remedies

Over the course of several years, Jane, a lady who was 45 years old, had been experiencing persistent pain in her lower back. In spite of the fact that she tried a number of conventional treatments, such as physical therapy and pain pills prescribed by a doctor, she only experienced short respite. After becoming dissatisfied with the adverse effects of her drugs, Jane looked for a method that was more natural in order to alleviate her discomfort.

Jane's integrative health practitioner recommended a customized herbal blend specifically designed to address inflammation and pain. The blend included turmeric for its potent anti-inflammatory properties, willow bark as a natural analgesic, and ginger to support overall joint health. Additionally, Jane was advised to incorporate a topical herbal salve made from arnica and St. John's Wort to apply directly to the affected area.

After six weeks of consistent use, Jane reported significant improvements in her pain levels and overall mobility. She was able to reduce her reliance on prescription medications and experienced fewer side effects. This case underscores the effectiveness of herbal remedies in managing chronic pain and highlights the importance of personalized treatment plans.

Case Study 2: Enhancing Cancer Treatment with Herbal Support

John, a 60-year-old man, was diagnosed with stage II colorectal cancer. As part of his treatment plan, he underwent surgery followed by chemotherapy. While the conventional treatments were necessary, John struggled with severe side effects, including nausea, fatigue, and a weakened immune system.

John's oncologist, who practiced integrative medicine, introduced an herbal support regimen to help mitigate the side effects of chemotherapy and enhance his overall well-being. The regimen included ginger and peppermint to combat nausea, milk thistle to support liver function, and astragalus to boost his immune system. Additionally, John was advised to drink green tea daily for its antioxidant properties.

Throughout his chemotherapy, John experienced significantly fewer side effects compared to his previous treatment cycles. His energy levels remained higher, and his immune system functioned more robustly, allowing him to maintain a better quality of life during a challenging time. This case illustrates how herbal remedies can be effectively integrated into conventional cancer treatments to support patient health.

Case Study 3: Addressing Anxiety and Insomnia with Herbal Therapies

Emily, a 32-year-old woman, had been struggling with anxiety and insomnia for several years. Conventional treatments, including anti-anxiety medications and sleep aids, provided some relief but also came with undesirable side effects, such as daytime drowsiness and dependency concerns.

Seeking a natural alternative, Emily consulted with an herbalist who recommended a comprehensive herbal treatment plan. The plan included valerian root and passionflower to promote relaxation and improve sleep quality, lemon balm to reduce anxiety, and ashwagandha to help manage stress. Emily was also encouraged to practice mindfulness meditation and incorporate aromatherapy using lavender essential oil into her bedtime routine.

After three months of following the herbal treatment plan, Emily reported significant improvements in both her anxiety and sleep patterns. She was able to discontinue her use of conventional sleep aids and experienced fewer anxiety episodes. This case highlights the potential of herbal remedies to provide effective and safer alternatives for managing mental health issues.

Case Study 4: Supporting Cardiovascular Health with Herbal Interventions

Mark, a 55-year-old man with a family history of heart disease, was diagnosed with hypertension and elevated cholesterol levels. His doctor prescribed medication to manage these conditions but also recommended lifestyle changes and herbal interventions to support cardiovascular health.

Mark's herbal regimen included hawthorn for its heart-strengthening properties, garlic to help lower cholesterol and blood pressure, and cayenne pepper to improve circulation. Additionally, he adopted a heart-healthy diet, increased his physical activity, and practiced stress-reduction techniques such as yoga.

Over six months, Mark's blood pressure and cholesterol levels improved significantly, and he was able to reduce his medication dosage under his doctor's supervision. His overall cardiovascular health benefited from the combined approach of conventional medicine and herbal support, demonstrating the value of an integrative treatment plan.

Case Study 5: Enhancing Digestive Health with Herbal Remedies

Lisa, a 40-year-old woman, experienced frequent digestive issues, including bloating, indigestion, and irritable bowel syndrome (IBS). Conventional treatments provided limited relief, prompting her to seek alternative options.

An integrative nutritionist recommended a blend of herbal remedies tailored to Lisa's digestive needs. This blend included peppermint and fennel to soothe the digestive tract, ginger to enhance digestion, and slippery elm to protect the gut lining. Lisa was also advised to incorporate probiotic-rich foods into her diet to support gut health.

After two months, Lisa reported a significant reduction in her digestive symptoms. She experienced less bloating and discomfort and noted an overall improvement in her digestive function. This case demonstrates the effectiveness of herbal remedies in managing digestive health issues and the importance of addressing the root causes of such conditions.

These real-life success stories exemplify the potential benefits of integrating herbal remedies with conventional medicine. Each case underscores the importance of personalized treatment plans, the role of healthcare providers in guiding patients through integrative approaches, and the need for ongoing monitoring and adjustment. By combining the strengths of both herbal and conventional medicine, patients can achieve improved health outcomes, enhanced quality of life, and a more holistic approach to their well-being. This integration not only honors the wisdom of traditional herbal practices but also leverages the advancements of modern medical science to provide comprehensive and effective healthcare solutions.

CHAPTER 9
Establishing a Natural Healing Lifestyle

9.1 Building a Natural Medicine Cabinet

Building a natural medicine cabinet is an essential step towards establishing a natural healing lifestyle. A well-stocked natural medicine cabinet allows you to address common health concerns promptly and effectively using herbal remedies, essential oils, and other natural products. This approach not only promotes self-reliance in managing health but also supports a holistic and preventive health philosophy. Below, we will explore the key components of a natural medicine cabinet, providing detailed insights into the herbs and remedies that should be included, their uses, and practical tips for storage and organization.

Essential Herbs and Their Uses

- **Chamomile (Matricaria chamomilla):** known for its relaxing effects, is a very useful herb. On a regular basis, it is utilized for the treatment of digestive disorders, anxiety, and insomnia. It is possible to treat skin irritations by consuming chamomile in the form of a tea, a tincture, or by applying it topically.
- **Echinacea (Echinacea purpurea):** is particularly well-known for the immune-enhancing characteristics that it possesses. At the beginning of the cold and flu season, it is frequently used to lessen the severity of symptoms and shorten their duration. The herb echinacea can be consumed in the form of a capsule, tincture, or tea.
- **Ginger (Zingiber officinale):** Ginger is a powerful anti-inflammatory and digestive aid. It is effective for treating nausea, motion sickness, and digestive discomfort. Ginger can be used fresh, dried, or as an essential oil.
- **Lavender (Lavandula angustifolia):** is a plant that is lauded for its ability to induce feelings of peace and relaxation. Those who suffer from stress, anxiety, or insomnia may find relief from its use. When it comes to aromatherapy and topical application, lavender essential oil is known to be extremely popular.
- **Peppermint (Mentha × piperita):** is a powerful digestive herb that has the ability to alleviate symptoms such as indigestion, gas, and bloating. Moreover, it is beneficial in treating headaches as well as muscle pain. Consuming peppermint in the form of a tea, tincture, or essential oil that has been diluted and administered topically are all viable options.
- **Turmeric (Curcuma longa):** Turmeric is well-known for the anti-inflammatory and antioxidant qualities that it possesses. Inflammation and discomfort are both managed with it, and it also helps to maintain general health. It is possible to consume turmeric in the form of a powder, pill, or tincture.

Essential Oils and Their Uses

* **Tea Tree Oil (Melaleuca alternifolia):** In addition to its powerful antibacterial characteristics, tea tree oil (Melaleuca alternifolia) is a useful treatment for a variety of skin conditions, including wounds, scrapes, and infections. Additionally, it can be utilized for the treatment of fungal infections and acne. It is imperative that tea tree oil be diluted prior to its application to the skin.
* **Eucalyptus Oil (Eucalyptus globulus):** Eucalyptus oil is excellent for respiratory issues. It can be used in steam inhalations to clear nasal congestion and soothe respiratory infections. It also has antiseptic properties for treating minor wounds.
* **Frankincense Oil (Boswellia sacra):** Frankincense oil is well-known for its ability to reduce inflammation and strengthen the immune system. It can be utilized for the treatment of skin conditions, relief of inflammation, and enhancement of immunological function. Aromatherapy is a common application for it, however it is also diluted for topical treatment.

Tinctures and Extracts

* **Valerian Root (Valeriana officinalis):** Valerian root tincture is effective for promoting sleep and reducing anxiety. It can be taken in small doses before bedtime to enhance sleep quality.
* **Milk Thistle (Silybum marianum):** A tincture made from milk thistle is beneficial to the liver's health and detoxification process. Those who have been exposed to toxins or those who are looking to improve the function of their liver can benefit from it.

Topical Remedies

* **Arnica (Arnica montana):** Arnica gel or cream is excellent for treating bruises, sprains, and muscle pain. It should not be applied to broken skin but is highly effective for reducing inflammation and pain in soft tissues.
* **Calendula (Calendula officinalis):** Calendula cream or ointment is perfect for soothing skin irritations, cuts, and burns. It has anti-inflammatory and antimicrobial properties, making it ideal for minor wounds and skin conditions.

Storage and Organization

A well-organized natural medicine cabinet ensures that remedies are easily accessible when needed. Here are some practical tips for setting up and maintaining your natural medicine cabinet:

* **Choose a Cool, Dark Location:** In order to preserve the effectiveness of herbs and essential oils, it is important to store them in a position that is both cool and dark. Avoid going to places that have a lot of humidity or direct sunshine.
* **Label Everything Clearly:** Clearly label all jars, bottles, and containers with the contents and date of preparation. This helps in keeping track of the shelf life and potency of each remedy.
* **Use Airtight Containers:** It is important to use airtight containers while storing dried herbs. To minimize moisture and air exposure, store dried herbs in airtight glass jars. In order to prevent light from damaging essential oils, it is recommended that they be stored in dark glass bottles.
* **Keep Tinctures and Extracts in Dropper Bottles:** Tinctures and extracts should be stored in dark dropper bottles for easy dosing and to protect them from light and air.
* **Create an Inventory List:** Maintain an inventory list of all the items in your natural medicine cabinet. This helps in keeping track of what you have and what needs to be replenished.

Example: Sarah, a mother of two who decided to transition her family to a more natural lifestyle. By building a natural medicine cabinet, Sarah was able to effectively manage common health issues that arose within her family. When her children caught a cold, she used echinacea and elderberry syrup to boost their immune systems and reduce symptoms. For her own stress and insomnia, Sarah relied on lavender and chamomile teas, which helped her relax and sleep better without the need for pharmaceuticals. When her husband experienced muscle pain after exercise, arnica gel provided quick relief. Sarah's natural medicine cabinet became an invaluable resource for her family's health, demonstrating the practical benefits of having a well-stocked supply of herbal remedies.

9.2 Sustainable and Ethical Sourcing of Herbs

Sustainable and ethical sourcing of herbs is a critical aspect of natural healing and herbal medicine. It ensures that the herbs we use are harvested in ways that protect the environment, support the livelihoods of local communities, and maintain the integrity and efficacy of the herbal products. Understanding and implementing sustainable practices in herb sourcing can contribute significantly to the conservation of biodiversity, the empowerment of indigenous populations, and the promotion of a more ethical approach to health and wellness.

One of the key principles of sustainable herb sourcing is minimizing the environmental impact of harvesting practices. This involves ensuring that herbs are collected in ways that do not deplete natural populations or damage ecosystems. Overharvesting can lead to the decline of plant species, disrupt habitats, and reduce biodiversity. Sustainable harvesting techniques include:

- **Rotational Harvesting:** This method involves rotating the areas from which herbs are collected, allowing plant populations to recover and regenerate between harvests. For example, wild ginseng is often harvested using rotational practices to ensure that the plants have adequate time to grow and reproduce.
- **Selective Harvesting:** Instead of removing entire plants, selective harvesting focuses on collecting only certain parts, such as leaves or flowers, while leaving the rest of the plant intact. This practice helps maintain the plant's health and its ability to continue growing. Harvesting only the outer leaves of a plant like aloe vera, for instance, allows the plant to continue thriving and producing more leaves.
- **Cultivation over Wildcrafting:** Where possible, cultivating herbs in controlled environments rather than wildcrafting can reduce pressure on wild populations. Cultivation also allows for better control over growing conditions and ensures a steady supply of high-quality herbs. Lavender, for example, is extensively cultivated to meet the high demand while protecting wild populations.

Ethical sourcing goes beyond environmental sustainability to include fair trade practices, transparency, and respect for indigenous knowledge. Ethical sourcing ensures that the people involved in growing, harvesting, and processing herbs are treated fairly and benefit from their work. Key aspects of ethical sourcing include:

- **Fair Wages and Working Conditions:** It is essential to ethical sourcing to make certain that workers are given fair salaries and that they are working in safe conditions. This contributes to the economic stability and well-being of the towns that are located in the area. Consumers can be assisted in identifying products that satisfy these standards through the use of fair trade certifications.

- **Respect for Indigenous Knowledge:** Many herbs used in modern herbal medicine have been part of indigenous cultures for centuries. Ethical sourcing involves recognizing and respecting this traditional knowledge and ensuring that indigenous communities benefit from the commercial use of their cultural heritage. For instance, the Hoodia plant, used by the San people of Southern Africa for its appetite-suppressing qualities, has become popular in weight loss products. Ethical sourcing would involve agreements that provide the San people with a share of the profits from Hoodia products.
- **Transparency and Traceability:** Ethical sourcing requires transparency about where and how herbs are sourced. This includes providing information about the origin of the herbs, the conditions under which they were grown and harvested, and the supply chain. Consumers can look for certifications such as FairWild, which ensures that wild-collected plants are harvested sustainably and ethically.

Example: Several companies and organizations are leading the way in sustainable and ethical herb sourcing. For example, the company Mountain Rose Herbs has implemented robust sustainability practices, including sourcing organic and fair trade-certified herbs, supporting reforestation projects, and ensuring ethical labor practices. Similarly, Traditional Medicinals, a producer of herbal teas, works directly with smallholder farmers and indigenous communities to source herbs ethically and sustainably, offering fair wages and investing in community development projects.

Consumers play a vital role in supporting sustainable and ethical herb sourcing. Here are some practical tips for making informed choices:

- **Research Brands and Certifications:** Look for companies that prioritize sustainability and ethical sourcing. Certifications like USDA Organic, Fair Trade, and FairWild provide assurance that the products meet high standards for environmental and social responsibility.
- **Support Local Growers:** Whenever possible, buy herbs from local farmers who use sustainable practices. Farmers' markets and community-supported agriculture (CSA) programs can be great sources of locally grown, sustainable herbs.
- **Ask Questions:** Don't hesitate to ask suppliers about their sourcing practices. Reputable companies will be transparent about where and how their herbs are sourced and processed.
- **Choose Organic:** Organic certification ensures that herbs are grown without synthetic pesticides and fertilizers, which can harm the environment and health. Organic farming practices also often include measures to protect soil health and biodiversity.

Sustainable and ethical sourcing of herbs is essential for preserving the environment, supporting local communities, and ensuring the quality and efficacy of herbal products. By adopting sustainable harvesting techniques, supporting fair trade practices, and promoting transparency in the supply chain, we can contribute to a more responsible and ethical herbal industry. As consumers, making informed choices and supporting companies that prioritize these values can drive positive change and help protect our planet's natural resources for future generations. Through conscious sourcing and consumption, we can enjoy the benefits of herbal medicine while honoring the earth and the people who cultivate its treasures.

9.3 Community and Support Networks

Community and support networks are fundamental components in establishing and maintaining a natural healing lifestyle. These networks provide essential resources, shared knowledge, emotional support, and a sense of belonging, all of which are crucial for individuals embarking on or continuing their journey into natural health practices. By fostering connections within a community, individuals can enhance their understanding of herbal remedies, share experiences, and receive guidance and encouragement from others with similar interests and goals.

A strong community provides a foundation of support and motivation for those pursuing a natural healing lifestyle. This sense of community can take many forms, from local herbal study groups and wellness clubs to online forums and social media groups dedicated to herbal medicine and natural healing practices. Within these communities, members can exchange knowledge about different herbs, share recipes, discuss experiences, and offer advice and support.

One of the key benefits of community involvement is the ability to learn from others' experiences. For example, a person new to using herbs for health might join a local herbal study group where more experienced members can provide practical tips on sourcing, preparing, and using herbs. This firsthand knowledge is invaluable and can significantly shorten the learning curve for beginners.

Additionally, communities can provide emotional support and encouragement, which are vital for sustaining long-term lifestyle changes. Knowing that others are facing similar challenges and celebrating similar successes can be incredibly motivating and help individuals stay committed to their natural healing journey.

There are various types of community and support networks that individuals can join to support their natural healing lifestyle:

- **Local Herbal Study Groups:** These groups typically meet regularly to discuss different herbs, their uses, and preparation methods. Members can bring their own experiences and questions, creating a collaborative learning environment.
- **Wellness Clubs and Workshops:** Many wellness centers and community organizations offer clubs and workshops focused on natural healing practices. These may include classes on herbal medicine, nutrition, yoga, and other holistic health practices.
- **Online Forums and Social Media Groups:** The internet provides a vast array of resources for connecting with others interested in natural healing. Online forums and social media groups allow individuals to share information, ask questions, and provide support regardless of geographical location.
- **Professional Associations:** Organizations such as the American Herbalists Guild (AHG) provide resources and networking opportunities for herbalists and those interested in herbal medicine. Membership often includes access to educational materials, conferences, and professional networks.
- **Community Gardens and Herbal Co-ops:** These initiatives allow individuals to grow herbs collectively, share harvests, and exchange knowledge about cultivation and uses. Community gardens are excellent for hands-on learning and building local connections.

Example: Consider the case of a community herbalist who starts a local herbal study group. The group meets biweekly and covers topics ranging from basic herbal preparations to advanced techniques like tincture making and herb cultivation. Over time, members form strong bonds, sharing personal stories of how herbal remedies have improved their health. One member, dealing with chronic stress, learns about the calming effects of adaptogenic herbs like ashwagandha and begins incorporating them into her routine with positive results. The group's collective knowledge and support empower her to make informed choices and stick with her new regimen.

Another example is an online forum dedicated to natural healing, where members from around the world discuss their experiences with different herbs, share success stories, and troubleshoot common issues. One participant, struggling with digestive problems, receives advice on using ginger and peppermint to alleviate symptoms. Encouraged by the support and detailed instructions from forum members, she tries these remedies and finds significant relief, contributing her success story back to the community.

Building a strong support network requires effort and engagement. Here are some steps to establish and maintain effective community and support networks:

- **Join Local Groups:** Look for local herbal study groups, wellness clubs, and community gardens. Participate actively by attending meetings, volunteering, and sharing your own knowledge and experiences.
- **Engage Online:** Join online forums and social media groups focused on herbal medicine and natural healing. Participate in discussions, ask questions, and offer your own insights. Online platforms can be particularly helpful for connecting with experts and accessing a wide range of perspectives.

- **Attend Workshops and Conferences:** Take part in workshops, seminars, and conferences that are associated with holistic health and herbal therapy. These events offer the chance to get knowledge from professionals, to have conversations with people who share similar interests, and to keep abreast of the most recent research and practices.
- **Create Your Own Group:** If local resources are limited, consider starting your own herbal study group or wellness club. Advertise through local community centers, social media, and word of mouth. Creating a space for people to come together and share their interest in natural healing can be incredibly rewarding.
- **Utilize Professional Associations:** Join professional organizations such as the American Herbalists Guild or the National Institute of Medical Herbalists. These associations offer valuable resources, networking opportunities, and professional development.
- **Foster Relationships:** Build strong, supportive relationships within your community. Offer help and support to others, and be open to receiving it in return. The strength of a community lies in the mutual respect and support of its members.

Community and support networks are indispensable for anyone committed to a natural healing lifestyle. They provide a wealth of knowledge, emotional support, and practical resources that can significantly enhance one's journey toward holistic health. By engaging with local groups, participating in online forums, attending workshops, and building strong relationships, individuals can create a robust support system that fosters growth, learning, and well-being. Whether through sharing personal experiences, offering advice, or simply being there to listen, the power of community cannot be overstated in the pursuit of natural healing and wellness.

9.4 Continuing Education and Resources for Natural Healing

In the ever-evolving field of natural healing, continuing education and access to reliable resources are vital for both practitioners and enthusiasts. Staying informed about the latest research, techniques, and trends not only enhances one's knowledge but also ensures the safe and effective use of herbal remedies. This commitment to lifelong learning fosters a deeper understanding of herbal medicine and supports the development of holistic health practices that are both current and evidence-based.

Continuing education in natural healing is essential for several reasons. First, it allows practitioners to stay updated on new discoveries and advancements in herbal medicine. This ongoing learning process ensures that their knowledge remains relevant and comprehensive. Second, it helps practitioners refine their skills, learn new techniques, and adopt best practices, thereby improving the quality of care they provide. Third, continuing education fosters a culture of critical thinking and scientific inquiry, encouraging practitioners to question assumptions, evaluate evidence, and make informed decisions.

For individuals seeking to deepen their understanding of natural healing, continuing education offers numerous benefits. It empowers them to make informed choices about their health, enhances their ability to manage common ailments naturally, and promotes overall well-being. By staying educated, individuals can also share their knowledge with others, contributing to a broader cultural shift towards holistic health practices.

1. **Formal Education Programs:** Enrolling in formal education programs, such as degrees or certifications in herbal medicine, naturopathy, or integrative health, provides a structured and comprehensive approach to learning. These programs often include coursework in botany, pharmacognosy, clinical skills, and ethics. Accredited institutions and professional organizations, such as the American Herbalists Guild (AHG) and the National Institute of Medical Herbalists (NIMH), offer certification programs that ensure rigorous standards and high-quality education.

2. **Workshops and Seminars:** Attending workshops and seminars is a great opportunity to learn practical skills and discuss natural healing trends. Practitioners and researchers who specialize in herbal formulation, plant identification, or holistic nutrition lead these events. Workshops and seminars offer hands-on learning and networking.

3. **Online Courses and Webinars:** Online courses and webinars offer flexible and accessible options for continuing education. Many reputable institutions and organizations provide online learning platforms that cover a wide range of topics in natural healing. These courses often include video lectures, reading materials, quizzes, and discussion forums. Examples include the Herbal Academy, which offers comprehensive online programs in herbal studies, and LearningHerbs, which provides practical, hands-on courses for all skill levels.

4. **Professional Conferences:** Professional conferences, such as the International Herbal Symposium or the AHG Symposium, bring together experts and practitioners from around the world to share their knowledge and research. These conferences offer a diverse array of presentations, workshops, and networking opportunities, allowing attendees to immerse themselves in the

latest trends and innovations in natural healing.

5. **Books and Journals:** Reading books and journals on herbal medicine and natural healing is an essential component of continuing education. Classic texts, such as "The Herbal Medicine-Maker's Handbook" by James Green or "Medical Herbalism" by David Hoffmann, provide foundational knowledge and practical guidance. Peer-reviewed journals, such as the "Journal of Herbal Medicine" and "Phytotherapy Research," publish the latest research findings and clinical studies, ensuring that practitioners stay informed about scientific advancements.

6. **Mentorship and Peer Networks:** Engaging in mentorship relationships and participating in peer networks can significantly enhance one's learning experience. Mentorship provides personalized guidance, feedback, and support from experienced practitioners. Peer networks, such as local herbal study groups or online communities, offer collaborative learning environments where members can share knowledge, discuss cases, and support each other's growth.

Example: Consider the case of a naturopathic practitioner who seeks to expand their knowledge of herbal remedies for mental health. By enrolling in an advanced online course on the subject, they gain access to in-depth lectures, case studies, and interactive discussions with experts in the field. This additional education enables the practitioner to integrate new treatment protocols into their practice, offering patients more effective and holistic options for managing conditions such as anxiety and depression.

Another example is a herbalist who attends an international conference focused on sustainable herbalism. Through workshops and networking sessions, they learn about innovative cultivation techniques, ethical sourcing practices, and emerging trends in herbal medicine. This experience not only enhances their professional knowledge but also inspires them to implement more sustainable practices in their own business, benefiting both their clients and the environment.

To make the most of continuing education resources, individuals should take a proactive and strategic approach:

- **Identify Learning Goals:** Clearly define what you want to achieve through continuing education. This could include mastering a specific herbal remedy, understanding the pharmacology of herbs, or staying updated on new research.
- **Research Options:** Explore the various education options available, from formal programs to informal workshops. Evaluate the credibility and reputation of the institutions and organizations offering these resources.
- **Create a Learning Plan:** Develop a structured plan that outlines your learning activities, timelines, and goals. This helps you stay focused and organized.
- **Engage Actively:** Participate actively in courses, workshops, and discussions. Ask questions, seek feedback, and apply what you learn to real-life situations.
- **Network and Collaborate:** Build relationships with peers, mentors, and experts in the field. Networking can provide valuable insights, support, and opportunities for collaboration.
- **Stay Updated:** Regularly read books, journals, and online resources to keep abreast of the latest developments in natural healing. Subscribe to newsletters, join professional associations, and attend conferences to stay connected to the broader community.

Continuing education and access to reliable

resources are essential for anyone committed to natural healing. By investing in lifelong learning, individuals can enhance their knowledge, refine their skills, and stay current with the latest advancements in herbal medicine. Whether through formal education programs, workshops, online courses, conferences, or reading, there are numerous opportunities to deepen one's understanding of natural healing. Embracing these resources empowers individuals to make informed health choices, provide better care, and contribute to the growing field of holistic health. By staying educated and connected, practitioners and enthusiasts alike can continue to evolve and thrive in their natural healing journey.

CHAPTER 10
The Future of Natural Healing

10.1 Emerging Trends in Herbal Medicine

Herbal medicine, a cornerstone of traditional healing practices, continues to evolve with the times, integrating modern scientific advancements and responding to contemporary health challenges. As society increasingly values natural and holistic approaches to health, several emerging trends are shaping the future of herbal medicine. These trends reflect a blend of tradition and innovation, enhancing the effectiveness, accessibility, and sustainability of herbal remedies.

One significant trend in herbal medicine is its growing integration with conventional medical practices. This trend is driven by a rising recognition of the benefits of holistic and complementary approaches in treating various health conditions. Integrative medicine combines the best of both worlds, using herbal remedies alongside conventional treatments to provide comprehensive care.

For instance, oncology centers are increasingly incorporating herbal supplements to help manage the side effects of chemotherapy. Herbs like ginger, used to alleviate nausea, and milk thistle, which supports liver function, are becoming standard adjuncts in cancer care protocols. This integration is supported by a growing body of clinical research validating the efficacy and safety of specific herbs when used in conjunction with conventional treatments.

Personalized medicine, tailored to an individual's genetic makeup, lifestyle, and specific health needs, is gaining traction in the field of herbal medicine. Advances in genomics and biotechnology enable practitioners to develop personalized herbal treatment plans that are more effective and precisely targeted.

For example, genetic testing can identify individuals who are more likely to benefit from certain herbs due to their unique metabolic profiles. This personalized approach ensures that patients receive the most suitable and effective herbal remedies, reducing the risk of adverse reactions and enhancing therapeutic outcomes.

As consumers become more environmentally conscious, the demand for sustainably and ethically sourced herbs is increasing. This trend emphasizes the importance of protecting biodiversity, supporting fair trade practices, and ensuring the long-term availability of medicinal plants.

Companies are adopting practices such as organic farming, wildcrafting with sustainable techniques, and supporting small-scale farmers. Certifications like FairWild and USDA Organic help consumers identify products that meet high standards of sustainability and ethical sourcing. This shift not only benefits the environment but also supports the livelihoods of communities involved in herb cultivation and harvesting.

Technology is playing a crucial role in advancing herbal medicine. From precision agriculture to digital health tools, technological innovations are enhancing the cultivation, processing, and utilization of herbs.

- **Precision Agriculture:** The use of drones, sensors, and data analytics in herb farming allows for precise monitoring of plant health, soil conditions, and environmental factors. This ensures optimal growing conditions, reduces the need for chemical inputs, and enhances the quality and yield of medicinal plants.
- **Digital Health Tools:** Mobile apps and wearable devices are providing new ways to track the effects of herbal remedies on health. Apps can remind users to take their herbal supplements, track symptoms, and provide personalized recommendations based on user data. Wearable devices can monitor physiological parameters like heart rate and sleep patterns, offering insights into the efficacy of herbal treatments.

The scientific community is increasingly recognizing the importance of rigorous research in herbal medicine. There is a growing number of clinical trials and studies aimed at understanding the mechanisms, efficacy, and safety of various herbs. This research is essential for integrating herbal medicine into mainstream healthcare and gaining acceptance among medical professionals.

For example, recent studies on turmeric have highlighted its potential in managing inflammatory conditions, leading to its incorporation into various therapeutic protocols. Similarly, research on adaptogenic herbs like ashwagandha and rhodiola is providing evidence for their use in managing stress and enhancing resilience.

The holistic health and wellness movement, which emphasizes the interconnectedness of physical, mental, and emotional well-being, is driving the popularity of herbal medicine. Consumers are increasingly seeking natural ways to support their overall health, prevent illness, and enhance their quality of life.

Herbal medicine is integral to this movement, offering solutions for stress management, sleep improvement, immune support, and more. Products like herbal teas, tinctures, and supplements are being marketed as part of a holistic lifestyle that includes mindfulness, nutrition, and physical activity.

The use of herbal remedies in mental health is another emerging trend. Herbs like St. John's Wort, valerian, and kava are being studied and used for their potential benefits in treating anxiety, depression, and sleep disorders. As mental health issues become more prevalent, the demand for natural and less invasive treatment options is increasing.

Integrative practitioners are incorporating these herbs into treatment plans, often in combination with conventional therapies, to enhance outcomes and reduce side effects. This holistic approach acknowledges the complex interplay between mind and body, offering a more comprehensive solution to mental health challenges.

8. Herbal Medicine for Chronic Conditions

Chronic conditions, such as diabetes, cardiovascular disease, and arthritis, are areas where herbal medicine is making significant inroads. Herbs with anti-inflammatory, antioxidant, and metabolic-regulating properties are being incorporated into treatment plans to manage symptoms and improve overall health.

For instance, herbs like cinnamon and fenugreek are used to support blood sugar regulation in diabetic patients. Hawthorn and garlic are recommended for cardiovascular health, while turmeric and boswellia are used to manage inflammation in arthritis.

Example: Consider the case of a holistic health clinic that integrates herbal medicine with conventional treatments. The clinic employs a team of practitioners, including naturopaths, herbalists, and medical doctors, who collaborate to create personalized treatment plans for their patients. This integrative approach has led to significant improvements in patient outcomes, particularly in managing chronic conditions and supporting mental health.

Another example is a community-supported agriculture (CSA) program focused on medicinal herbs. This initiative allows consumers to buy shares in a local herb farm, receiving regular deliveries of fresh, sustainably grown herbs. This model supports local farmers, promotes sustainable agriculture, and provides consumers with high-quality, fresh herbs for their health needs.

The future of herbal medicine is being shaped by several emerging trends that reflect a blend of tradition and innovation. Increased integration with conventional medicine, personalized approaches, sustainable sourcing, technological advancements, rigorous research, holistic health, mental health applications, and the management of chronic conditions are all contributing to the evolving landscape of herbal medicine. These trends highlight the potential of herbal remedies to enhance health and well-being in a holistic, sustainable, and scientifically validated manner. By staying informed and embracing these trends, practitioners and consumers alike can continue to benefit from the rich traditions and modern advancements in herbal medicine.

10.2 The Role of Technology in Natural Health

The integration of technology into the field of natural health is transforming how we approach wellness, making holistic practices more accessible, effective, and personalized. From advanced diagnostic tools to digital health platforms, technology is enhancing the ways we understand and utilize natural healing methods. This evolution is fostering a more integrative approach to health care, where traditional herbal remedies and modern medical advancements work hand-in-hand to promote overall well-being.

One of the most significant contributions of technology to natural health is the proliferation of digital health platforms and mobile applications. These tools provide users with convenient access to a wealth of information on natural remedies, wellness practices, and personalized health management.

- **Health Tracking Apps:** These applications allow users to monitor various aspects of their health, such as sleep patterns, physical activity, and dietary habits. By integrating with wearable devices, these apps can track physiological data in real-time, providing insights into how different lifestyle choices impact overall health. For example, an app like MyFitnessPal can help users log their food intake and track their nutrient consumption, while also suggesting dietary adjustments to meet specific health goals.
- **Telemedicine Platforms:** Telemedicine has revolutionized access to health care, enabling consultations with healthcare providers through video calls, chat, and email. This technology is particularly beneficial for individuals seeking guidance on natural health practices from experts who may not be geographically

accessible. For instance, platforms like HealthTap or Doctor on Demand offer virtual consultations with naturopathic doctors and herbalists, allowing patients to receive personalized advice and treatment plans.

Wearable devices, such as fitness trackers and smartwatches, have become invaluable tools in monitoring and promoting natural health. These devices provide real-time data on various health metrics, enabling users to make informed decisions about their wellness routines.

- **Fitness Trackers:** Devices like Fitbit and Garmin track physical activity, heart rate, sleep quality, and more. By providing continuous feedback, these trackers help users stay motivated and make necessary adjustments to their lifestyle. For example, tracking sleep patterns can highlight the impact of certain herbal supplements, like valerian root or melatonin, on improving sleep quality.
- **Smartwatches:** Smartwatches such as the Apple Watch offer advanced health monitoring features, including electrocardiograms (ECGs), blood oxygen level tracking, and irregular heart rhythm notifications. These capabilities allow users to monitor their cardiovascular health closely and take preventive measures using natural remedies and lifestyle changes.

Artificial Intelligence (AI) and Big Data are playing increasingly prominent roles in natural health by enabling the analysis of vast amounts of health data to identify patterns and make predictions. These technologies are helping to personalize health care and improve the efficacy of natural treatments.

- **Personalized Health Recommendations:** AI-driven platforms can analyze individual health data, including genetic information, to provide personalized recommendations for diet, exercise, and herbal supplements. For instance, the app Nutrigenomix uses genetic testing to offer tailored nutritional advice, helping users optimize their diet based on their genetic predispositions.
- **Research and Development:** Big Data is accelerating research in herbal medicine by allowing researchers to analyze extensive datasets to uncover the therapeutic potential of various herbs. This analysis can lead to the discovery of new herbal remedies and the development of more effective treatment protocols.

Virtual Reality (VR) and Augmented Reality (AR) are innovative technologies that are beginning to find applications in natural health, particularly in education and therapeutic practices.

- **Educational Tools:** VR and AR can create immersive learning experiences for students and practitioners of herbal medicine. For example, virtual herb gardens and interactive AR applications can help users identify plants, learn about their medicinal properties, and understand their uses in a more engaging and intuitive way.
- **Therapeutic Applications:** VR is being used in mental health therapy to create calming and meditative environments that aid in stress reduction and relaxation. For instance, VR programs designed to simulate nature walks or guided meditations can enhance the therapeutic effects of natural health practices.

Precision agriculture, driven by advancements in technology, is transforming the cultivation of medicinal herbs. This approach uses data analytics, drones, and sensors to optimize farming practices, ensuring the sustainable and efficient production of high-quality herbs.

- **Drones and Sensors:** The use of drones

that are fitted with multispectral sensors allows for the monitoring of the health of herb crops, the detection of insect infestations, and the evaluation of the conditions of the soil. The use of toxic chemicals can be reduced and organic farming methods can be encouraged through the utilization of this technology, which enables farmers to make decisions regarding irrigation, fertilization, and pest management based on data-driven information.

- **Data Analytics:** By analyzing data collected from various sources, farmers can predict optimal harvest times, improve crop yields, and enhance the potency of medicinal herbs. This precision in farming ensures that the herbs used in natural health practices are of the highest quality.

Blockchain technology is emerging as a powerful tool for ensuring transparency and traceability in the herbal supply chain. This technology can help consumers and practitioners verify the authenticity and quality of herbal products.

- **Supply Chain Transparency:** Blockchain can track the journey of herbs from farm to consumer, providing detailed information about their cultivation, harvesting, and processing. This transparency helps ensure that herbs are sourced ethically and sustainably.
- **Quality Assurance:** Blockchain can be used to verify the purity and potency of herbal products, ensuring that they meet high standards of quality. This technology can help build consumer trust and confidence in natural health products.

Example: A notable example of technology enhancing natural health is the platform Gaia Herbs. Gaia Herbs uses precision agriculture techniques to cultivate high-quality herbs, ensuring the purity and potency of their products. They employ drone technology to monitor crop health and use blockchain to provide transparency about their sourcing and production processes.

Another example is the use of AI in the development of personalized herbal supplements. Companies like Sun Genomics use microbiome analysis to create custom probiotics tailored to an individual's gut health. By analyzing genetic data and health metrics, these companies can formulate supplements that address specific health needs, enhancing the effectiveness of natural remedies.

The role of technology in natural health is multifaceted, offering numerous advancements that enhance the accessibility, effectiveness, and sustainability of herbal medicine. Digital health platforms, wearable devices, AI, VR, precision agriculture, and blockchain technology are all contributing to a more integrated and personalized approach to wellness. By embracing these technological innovations, practitioners and consumers can leverage the best of both traditional and modern medicine, fostering a holistic and informed approach to health. As technology continues to evolve, its integration with natural health practices promises to further revolutionize the way we understand, use, and benefit from herbal remedies.

10.3 Innovations and Research in Natural Healing

The field of natural healing is undergoing a transformative phase, driven by a combination of cutting-edge research and innovative practices. This evolution is expanding our understanding of traditional remedies and introducing new methods that enhance the efficacy and accessibility of natural treatments. The integration of scientific research with traditional knowledge is paving the way for more effective, evidence-based approaches to health and wellness.

Recent years have seen a significant increase in scientific research focused on understanding the biochemical properties and therapeutic potential of various herbs. This research is crucial for validating the efficacy of traditional remedies and integrating them into mainstream healthcare.

- **Phytochemistry:** Advances in phytochemistry have enabled researchers to isolate and study the active compounds in medicinal plants. Understanding these compounds' mechanisms of action helps in determining how they contribute to health and healing. For example, curcumin, the active compound in turmeric, has been extensively studied for its anti-inflammatory and antioxidant properties. These studies have led to the development of standardized curcumin supplements used to treat conditions like arthritis and inflammatory bowel disease.

- **Clinical Trials:** In order to determine whether or not herbal medicines are safe and effective, it is necessary to conduct scientifically rigorous clinical trials. Clinical trials of this kind give the evidence that is required to support the utilization of these treatments in clinical settings. Echinacea, for example, has been shown to be helpful in lowering the duration and intensity of the common cold, which has led to its broad acceptance and use as an immune booster. This has been proved through a series of clinical investigations.

Natural healing is undergoing a revolutionary change as a result of a ground-breaking discovery that involves the incorporation of genomics technologies. Through the use of personalized medicine, treatments can be tailored to an individual based on their genetic composition, lifestyle, and health history. This makes it feasible to produce natural medicines that are more precise and successful.

- **Nutrigenomics:** This branch of genomics studies the interaction between nutrition and genes. It aims to understand how different foods and nutrients affect gene expression and health outcomes. By analyzing an individual's genetic profile, nutrigenomics can provide personalized dietary recommendations that optimize health and prevent disease. For example, someone with a genetic predisposition to inflammation might benefit from a diet rich in anti-inflammatory herbs like ginger and turmeric.

- **Pharmacogenomics:** This field examines how genetic variations affect individual responses to medications, including herbal remedies. By understanding these genetic differences, practitioners can predict which patients are likely to benefit from specific herbs and at what dosages. This personalized approach minimizes adverse effects and enhances therapeutic outcomes.

Innovations in delivery systems are enhancing the bioavailability and efficacy of natural remedies. Traditional forms of administration, such as teas and tinctures, are being complemented by advanced technologies that ensure optimal absorption and effectiveness.

- **Nanotechnology:** Nanotechnology involves manipulating substances at the molecular or atomic level. In natural healing, nanotechnology is used to create nano-sized particles of herbal compounds, improving their solubility and absorption. For instance, nano-curcumin is a form of curcumin with significantly enhanced bioavailability, making it more effective in reducing inflammation and pain.

- **Liposome Technology:** Liposomes are tiny vesicles that can encapsulate active compounds, protecting them from degradation and enhancing their absorption. Liposomal delivery systems are used to improve the bioavailability of herbal extracts, such as liposomal vitamin C and liposomal CBD, providing more consistent and potent effects.

The development of integrative healthcare models is another significant innovation in natural healing. These models combine conventional medicine with complementary therapies, providing a holistic approach to patient care.

- **Functional Medicine:** Functional medicine addresses the root causes of disease rather than just treating symptoms. It incorporates natural remedies, nutrition, and lifestyle modifications into personalized treatment plans. For example, a functional medicine approach to treating chronic fatigue syndrome might include dietary changes, stress management techniques, and herbal adaptogens like ashwagandha and rhodiola.
- **Integrative Oncology:** Integrative oncology combines conventional cancer treatments with supportive natural therapies to enhance patient outcomes and quality of life. Herbal supplements, acupuncture, and nutritional support are used to manage side effects and support overall health during cancer treatment. Research in this field has shown that integrative approaches can improve symptom management, reduce treatment side effects, and enhance patients' emotional well-being.

Digital health and telemedicine are making natural healing more accessible and convenient for patients. These technologies provide platforms for remote consultations, personalized treatment plans, and continuous health monitoring.

- **Telehealth Platforms:** Telehealth platforms allow patients to consult with naturopathic doctors and herbalists from the comfort of their homes. This accessibility is particularly beneficial for those living in remote areas or with limited mobility. For example, platforms like Wellevate and Fullscript offer telehealth consultations and direct delivery of herbal supplements.
- **Health Monitoring Apps:** Mobile apps that track health metrics, such as diet, physical activity, and sleep, help individuals monitor their progress and make informed decisions about their health. Apps like MyFitnessPal and Cronometer allow users to log their food intake and track nutrient consumption, integrating this data with personalized health recommendations.

The proliferation of educational resources and online communities is empowering individuals to take control of their health and wellness. Access to accurate information and support networks is crucial for making informed decisions about natural healing.

- **Online Courses and Webinars:** Many institutions and organizations offer online courses and webinars on various aspects of natural healing. These educational resources provide in-depth knowledge and practical skills for both practitioners and enthusiasts. The Herbal Academy, for example, offers comprehensive online programs in herbal studies, covering everything from basic herb identification to advanced clinical applications.
- **Online Communities:** Social media platforms and forums create spaces for individuals to share experiences, ask questions, and receive support from like-minded people. These communities foster a sense of belonging and encourage the exchange of knowledge and resources. Platforms like Reddit's r/

herbalism and Facebook groups dedicated to natural healing provide valuable insights and peer support.

Sustainability and ethical sourcing are becoming central to the practice of natural healing. Ensuring that herbs are sourced responsibly protects the environment and supports the communities involved in their cultivation.

- **Organic Farming**: Organic farming practices avoid the use of synthetic pesticides and fertilizers, promoting soil health and biodiversity. Herbs grown organically are free from harmful chemicals, ensuring their purity and potency. Companies like Gaia Herbs and Mountain Rose Herbs prioritize organic and sustainable farming practices, setting a standard for the industry.
- **Fair Trade Practices**: Fair trade certifications ensure that farmers and workers receive fair wages and work in safe conditions. Supporting fair trade products helps improve the livelihoods of those involved in herb production and promotes ethical business practices. Fair-Wild is a certification that guarantees sustainable and equitable wild plant harvesting, supporting both environmental and social sustainability.

Example: Consider the advancements in the use of adaptogens, a class of herbs that help the body adapt to stress. Recent research has focused on understanding the mechanisms of adaptogens like ashwagandha, rhodiola, and holy basil. Studies have shown that these herbs can modulate the stress response, improve energy levels, and enhance cognitive function. These findings have led to the development of targeted adaptogenic supplements designed to support mental and physical resilience.

Another example is the use of digital health platforms to deliver personalized herbal medicine. Companies like Sun Genomics use microbiome analysis to create custom probiotics tailored to an individual's gut health. By integrating genetic data and health metrics, these platforms provide personalized recommendations that optimize gut health and overall wellness.

Innovations and research in natural healing are driving the field forward, blending traditional wisdom with modern science to create more effective and accessible treatments. Advances in phytochemistry, genomics, delivery systems, integrative healthcare models, digital health, education, and sustainability are transforming how we understand and practice natural healing. By staying informed and embracing these innovations, practitioners and individuals can harness the full potential of natural remedies, contributing to a more holistic and scientifically grounded approach to health and wellness.

Conclusion

The exploration of natural healing has revealed an intricate tapestry woven from centuries-old traditions and cutting-edge scientific advancements. This journey through the various chapters has highlighted the significance of understanding the historical context, the body's innate healing processes, and the synergistic relationship between mind, body, and spirit. Furthermore, the comprehensive discussion on the power of nutrition, the role of herbs, and the importance of personalized herbal blends has emphasized the multi-faceted approach necessary for holistic wellness. In this concluding chapter, we synthesize these insights, underscoring the profound potential of natural healing in contemporary healthcare and the transformative impact it can have on individual and collective well-being.

Natural healing, grounded in ancient wisdom, continues to thrive in the modern era by embracing scientific validation and technological innovation. The historical context and evolution of herbal medicine demonstrate that these practices are not static but dynamically evolving. Traditional remedies, once passed down orally or through simple manuscripts, are now subjected to rigorous scientific scrutiny. This validation process has not only affirmed the efficacy of many herbal treatments but also dispelled myths, ensuring that what we adopt in contemporary practice is both safe and effective.

The integration of modern technology, such as precision agriculture and blockchain, has revolutionized the way we cultivate, process, and distribute herbal products. These advancements ensure sustainability, quality, and traceability, addressing concerns about environmental impact and ethical sourcing. The synergy between ancient practices and modern innovations exemplifies a holistic approach that respects the past while embracing the future.

The holistic approach to health underscores the interconnectedness of mind, body, and spirit. This triad forms the foundation of well-being, where imbalances in one aspect can affect the others. The role of mind, body, and spirit in wellness is pivotal, as it highlights the necessity of addressing all dimensions of health. For instance, stress and anxiety, predominantly psychological issues, can manifest physically as digestive problems or weakened immunity. Conversely, physical ailments can lead to emotional distress and spiritual disconnection.

Herbal medicine, with its rich array of therapeutic properties, offers remedies that cater to these interconnected aspects. Adaptogens like ashwagandha and rhodiola help the body adapt to stress, simultaneously supporting mental clarity and emotional resilience. Calming herbs such as chamomile and lavender promote relaxation and improve sleep, addressing both mental and physical health. By incorporating herbs that support all facets of health, natural healing practices foster a comprehensive approach to wellness.

Nutrition plays a crucial role in natural healing, acting as the cornerstone of health. The discussions on macronutrients, micronutrients, and superfoods have underscored the importance of a balanced diet rich in essential nutrients. Herbs and natural remedies are integral to this nutritional approach, providing additional benefits that enhance overall health.

Superfoods, such as spirulina, chia seeds, and turmeric, are celebrated for their high nutrient density and medicinal properties. These foods support various bodily functions, from boosting immunity to reducing inflammation. The concept of detoxification further illustrates the interplay between nutrition and natural healing. By incorporating herbs like milk thistle and dandelion, which support liver function, detoxification processes are enhanced, promoting the elimination of toxins and improving overall vitality.

Herbs are at the heart of natural healing, offering a diverse array of therapeutic benefits. The comprehensive coverage of key herbs, such as chamomile, echinacea, ginger, and lavender, has provided insights into their specific uses and mechanisms of action. These herbs are not only effective in treating specific ailments but also in maintaining general health and preventing disease.

The practice of creating custom herbal blends exemplifies the personalized approach central to natural healing. By tailoring blends to individual needs, practitioners can address specific health concerns more effectively. This customization considers factors such as the patient's constitution, existing health conditions, and lifestyle, ensuring that the herbal treatments are both appropriate and potent.

Sustainability and ethical sourcing are critical to the integrity of natural healing practices. The growing awareness of environmental impact and social responsibility has led to the adoption of sustainable harvesting techniques, fair trade practices, and transparency in the herbal supply chain. These measures ensure that the benefits of herbal medicine extend beyond individual health to encompass ecological and community well-being.

Ethical sourcing also respects the traditional knowledge of indigenous communities, acknowledging their contributions and ensuring that they benefit from the commercialization of their heritage. Companies adhering to certifications like Fair-Wild and USDA Organic set standards for quality and sustainability, fostering trust and accountability in the industry.

Community and support networks are indispensable for those pursuing a natural healing lifestyle. These networks provide shared knowledge, emotional support, and a sense of belonging, crucial for maintaining long-term health practices. Whether through local herbal study groups, online forums, or professional associations, engaging with a community enhances one's understanding and application of natural remedies.

Continuing education is equally vital, ensuring that practitioners and enthusiasts stay updated on the latest research, techniques, and innovations. Access to reliable resources, such as workshops, online courses, and professional journals, fosters a culture of lifelong learning. This commitment to education empowers individuals to make informed decisions about their health and contribute to the broader field of natural healing.

The future of natural healing is promising, marked by emerging trends and innovations that enhance its effectiveness and accessibility. The integration of technology, such as digital health platforms, wearable devices, and AI-driven personalized medicine, is transforming how we approach natural health. These advancements provide more precise, data-driven insights, enabling personalized treatment plans that optimize health outcomes.

Research and clinical trials continue to validate the efficacy of herbal remedies, bridging the gap between traditional knowledge and scientific evidence. This research is crucial for integrating natural healing into mainstream healthcare, fostering acceptance and utilization by medical professionals.

Innovations in herbal medicine are expanding the possibilities of natural healing. Advanced delivery systems, such as nanotechnology and liposomal encapsulation, enhance the bioavailability and potency of herbal compounds. These innovations ensure that the therapeutic benefits of herbs are maximized, providing more effective treatments.

Integrative healthcare models, such as functional medicine and integrative oncology, exemplify the holistic approach central to natural healing. These models combine conventional and complementary therapies, addressing the root causes of disease and promoting overall well-being. By incorporating natural remedies into comprehensive treatment plans, practitioners can offer more effective and personalized care.

Technology plays a crucial role in the evolution of natural health practices. From digital health platforms that provide easy access to information and consultations to precision agriculture that ensures the sustainable cultivation of medicinal herbs, technology is enhancing every aspect of natural healing. Wearable devices and health tracking apps empower individuals to monitor their health in real-time, making informed decisions about their wellness routines. AI and Big Data are driving personalized health recommendations, ensuring that treatments are tailored to individual needs.

Blockchain technology ensures transparency and traceability in the herbal supply chain, building consumer trust and guaranteeing the quality and authenticity of herbal products. Virtual Reality (VR) and Augmented Reality (AR) are creating immersive educational tools and therapeutic applications, enhancing learning and treatment experiences.

The field of natural healing is at an exciting juncture, where tradition meets innovation, and science validates age-old wisdom. This convergence offers a holistic, effective, and sustainable approach to health and wellness. By embracing the historical context of herbal medicine, understanding the interconnectedness of mind, body, and spirit, and integrating modern technological advancements, we can unlock the full potential of natural healing.

The commitment to sustainable and ethical practices ensures that we protect the environment and support the communities involved in herbal cultivation. Community support and continuing education empower individuals to make informed decisions about their health, fostering a culture of lifelong learning and shared knowledge.

As we look to the future, the role of technology, ongoing research, and innovative practices will continue to shape the field of natural healing. This evolution promises to enhance the accessibility, effectiveness, and integration of natural remedies into mainstream healthcare, offering a holistic approach that promotes overall well-being.

Made in United States
Orlando, FL
07 October 2024

52503822R00065